PREVENTING
LYME
& Other Tick-Borne Diseases

ALEXIS CHESNEY, ND

Storey Publishing

The mission of Storey Publishing is to serve our customers by
publishing practical information that encourages
personal independence in harmony with the environment.

EDITED BY Carleen Madigan, Nancy Ringer, and Sarah Guare
COVER DESIGN BY Michaela Jebb
BOOK DESIGN BY Michaela Jebb and Erin Dawson
INDEXED BY Christine R. Lindemer, Boston Road Communications

COVER PHOTOGRAPHY BY mrs/Getty Images
LYME RASH ID PHOTOGRAPHY BY © anakopa/iStock.com, 1 t.l.; Originally printed as reference for
"Diagnostic challenges of early Lyme disease: Lessons from a community case series," by John
Aucott et al. *BMC Infectious Diseases* 9, 79 (2009). www.researchgate.net/publication/26257313.
Licensed via the CC BY 2.0., 2 b.r.; © dennisjacobsen/stock.adobe.com, 1 b.r.; © imageBROKER/
Alamy Stock Photo, 1 t.r.; © JerryCallaghan/iStock.com, 1 b.l.; © Jaroslav Moravcik/stock.adobe
.com, 2 t.r.; Mikael Häggström/Wikimedia Commons, 2 t.l.; Originally printed as reference for
"Bullous Lyme disease" by Jeffrey B. Tiger, Marshall A. Guill III, and M. Shane Champman. *Journal of
the American Academy of Dermatology* 71, no. 4 (2014). www.sciencedirect.com/science/article/pii/
S0190962214013917. Licensed via the CC BY-NC-ND 4.0., 2 b.l.; © Tramper2/stock.adobe.com, 1 m.r.
ILLUSTRATIONS BY Beverly Duncan, except page 78 by Ilona Sherratt
RANGE MAPS BY Ilona Sherratt
Life cycle diagram on page 30 based on an illustration created by the Centers for Disease Control and
Prevention (www.cdc.gov/lyme/transmission/blacklegged.html)

**This publication is intended to provide educa-
tional information on the covered subject. It is
not intended to take the place of personalized
medical counseling, diagnosis, and treatment
from a trained health professional.**

Storey Publishing
210 MASS MoCA Way
North Adams, MA 01247
storey.com

Printed in the United States by Versa Press
10 9 8 7 6 5 4 3 2 1

Library of Congress Cataloging-in-Publication
Data on file

To all of my patients
Thank you for the honor of inviting me to
walk with you on your healing journeys.

And to my grandmother "Nani"
Thank you for your love and inspiration. I would not
be where I am today had it not been for you.

CONTENTS

FOREWORD

Why It's Important to Protect Yourself from Tick-Borne Diseases

OVER THE LAST SEVERAL DECADES, tick-borne diseases (TBD) have been slowly spreading across the United States and the rest of the world, adversely affecting the lives of millions of people. In this country, all 50 states have reported cases of Lyme disease, and the numbers keep increasing. During the last 20 years, there has been a 320 percent increase in U.S. counties reporting ticks containing Lyme disease, as well as an alarming threefold increase in vector-borne disease cases overall. Confirming these public health reports, Quest Laboratories recently reported close to a doubling of positive Lyme testing among those being screened in 2018. These rising numbers do not account for those never screened, those who are tested but whose results show a false negative for Lyme (due to the insensitivity of the testing), or those who are never screened for associated co-infections present in the ticks.

Co-infection of ticks is now the rule, not the exception, and up to 85 percent of those with Lyme disease have been exposed to other pathogens in ticks. And transmission can happen rapidly: Powassan virus can be transmitted within 15 minutes of a tick bite, rickettsial infections can be transmitted within 10 minutes, and the relapsing fever borrelia, *Borrelia hermsii*, can be transmitted within just 5 minutes.

The symptoms of many of these co-infections can mimic those of Lyme. Even with early antibiotic treatment, they can have long-term disabling effects, adversely affecting the quality of your life and impairing your ability to work and be a productive member of society. Co-infections are potentially fatal in the young and elderly, especially in those with impaired immune system functioning.

Tick-borne infections can also mimic other chronic debilitating conditions, including chronic fatigue syndrome/myalgic encephalomyelitis, fibromyalgia, autoimmune diseases like rheumatoid arthritis or multiple sclerosis, and even autism or Alzheimer's disease. Tick-borne infections combined with environmental toxins have been reported in the medical literature to potentially play a role in all of these diseases. In fact, after seeing more than 13,000 chronically ill individuals with Lyme and TBD during the past 30 years, I am convinced that tick-borne infections are at the root of many unexplained symptoms and illnesses. In searching for answers for my sick and suffering patients, I have found up to 16 reasons why people may remain ill. I call this MSIDS — multiple infectious disease syndrome — and this model accounts for how tick-borne infections, along with overlapping sources of inflammation and their downstream effects, can lead to chronic illness.

Proper prevention is crucial, and the measures Dr. Chesney outlines in this book will certainly help save lives and prevent unnecessary suffering. There is no reason to tempt fate. Every time you go outside, use the tick-prevention measures discussed in this book. A small tick can cause long-lasting health issues that keep you from living life to the fullest. You will be well served to be mindful of this spreading epidemic, follow Dr. Chesney's advice, and protect yourself and your loved ones accordingly.

> **—RICHARD HOROWITZ, MD,** *New York Times* bestselling
> author of *Why Can't I Get Better?* and *How Can I Get Better?*

PREFACE

MY GRANDMOTHER HAD RHEUMATIC FEVER as a child and, as a result, she suffered from heart-related complications her whole life. Growing up, I spent a lot of time visiting her at the hospital. This was the same hospital where my aunt worked, where I later volunteered, and where I returned to work as a nurse extender the year after I graduated from college. This meant that I worked on a medical-surgical floor supporting the nurses as I drew blood, took vital signs, and monitored the telemetry, as well as providing comfort care to patients. At the same time, I was preparing for the MCAT (Medical College Admission Test).

I really loved the hospital but felt there was something missing. I found myself constantly thinking about what had happened to all these patients before they became so ill. What had led them to need heart surgery and chronic medications? I started reading Dr. Andrew Weil's books and learning more about natural therapies. The idea that the body had an inherent capacity to heal itself resonated strongly with me. Preventing heart disease — the leading cause of death in the United States — through diet, exercise, and lifestyle changes made sense to me. This shift in perspective led me to enter school to begin training as a naturopathic doctor in Bridgeport, Connecticut, instead of becoming a conventional allopathic doctor.

After I began practicing as a naturopath, I began to look back at my grandmother's condition differently. Her heart disease was caused by a bacterium — group A streptococcus — that she had been exposed to when she was 8 years old. Penicillin had not yet been discovered to treat her infection. She developed rheumatic fever, which caused endocarditis, an inflammation of the heart and its valves. Later, she was one of the first people to be given a replacement valve, and that saved her life. Fortunately, with the help of medication, she lived to the age of 77. I am forever grateful to the interventions of the allopathic world for this. However, I found myself wondering: If naturopathic medicine, especially herbal medicine, had been available when she was a child, could it have prevented the infection from ever affecting her heart? Perhaps my personal experience with my grandmother and my relationship to her illness planted a seed. When I began to work with people whose suffering was caused by a different bacterium — the one that causes Lyme disease — this seed would germinate into the work I do today.

In fact, my journey with Lyme disease started during my naturopathic medical education in Connecticut when a friend of mine came down with an illness that was discovered to be Lyme disease. Luckily she received treatment from a Lyme-literate medical doctor. The complexity of symptoms and the challenge to get proper treatment inspired me to learn more. In 2010, I completed an internship with Richard Horowitz, MD, a well-known expert in Lyme and tick-borne diseases (TBD). It was a gift to glean all the information I possibly could from him regarding the diagnosis and treatment of these conditions. My internship with Dr. Horowitz equipped me to answer my calling to work with those with Lyme and TBD. I had just begun practicing at Sojourns Community Health Clinic, a rural integrative clinic in Westminster, Vermont, with a new passion for detecting Lyme disease and with resources to test for and treat it. At the time, I had not realized that I arrived on the front line in the Lyme epidemic in Vermont in 2010. Patients told me stories about conventional physicians denying that there were ticks in Vermont, let alone Lyme disease. Soon after, in 2013, Vermont became the top state in the nation for Lyme disease incidence.

Currently, my patient population ranges from patients with early to late Lyme disease and from those who have one easily treated infection to others who have complex chronic illness. I see patients with the classic bull's-eye rash (known as erythema migrans) that is diagnostic for Lyme disease who do very well with prompt comprehensive treatment and go on living symptom-free. However, I mainly work with patients who have delayed proper treatment of Lyme disease because of the lack of knowledge about the disease, misdiagnosis, or confounding complex chronic illness. More frequent, more severe, and more numerous symptoms correlate with longer, more complex treatments. The longer the delay of comprehensive treatment, and the more tick-borne diseases (or coinfections) involved, the longer and more elaborate the treatment must be. I have worked with many people who have struggled on their healing journeys. I have seen people improve and many become symptom-free.

It has been an honor to witness the stories of hundreds who have been affected by the Lyme epidemic, to hold space for each patient as a whole person with an innate ability to heal, to guide the patient in testing and treatment options, and to observe the healing process. It is not unusual for someone to undergo an identity crisis and experience a range of emotions associated with the process. When people trust their bodies, their intuition, their practitioners, their treatment, and their support system, I see healing happen.

During, and especially after, treatment, I emphasize the importance of tick bite prevention. As with Lyme treatment, I individualize patients' preventive plans based on their profile for tick contact. Unfortunately, overcoming Lyme disease once does not protect you from further exposures. And if you have not had Lyme, at the rate this epidemic is progressing, it may be more accurate to say you haven't contracted it *yet*.

I'm writing this book to promote awareness of prevention strategies. Without an effective vaccine, accurate testing, or simple effective treatment, each of us must do our part to educate ourselves and each other in order to stop the Lyme disease epidemic. My hope is that I may empower a movement to halt the spread of Lyme and TBD through prevention. Prevention is the best cure!

Introduction

LYME DISEASE IS THE MOST COMMON vector-borne illness in the United States. A vector is an organism, such as a tick, that transmits a pathogen like *Borrelia burgdorferi* (which causes Lyme disease) from one organism to another. There are more than 300,000 new cases of Lyme disease diagnosed each year. The number of cases has increased to about 25 times the amount reported in 1982 when surveillance of the disease began. More than half of cases occur in children. As the incidence of Lyme disease has increased in the Northeast, so has the number of patients I see. In 2015, the Centers for Disease Control and Prevention (CDC) showed a 320 percent rise in the incidence of Lyme disease in the northeastern United States and a 250 percent rise in the north-central states. This was the second year (2013 was the first) that Vermont had the highest incidence of Lyme disease in the nation. To change the tide, radical education on the prevention of Lyme disease is critical. This book will provide practical strategies that everyone — from the weekend outdoor enthusiast to the professional farmer — can use. Fortunately, you can take many steps to prevent Lyme and tick-borne disease, including managing the tick population in your yard, preventing ticks from getting on you, and treating tick bites promptly and properly if and when they happen.

Naturopathic Medicine

I am a naturopathic physician, which means I treat Lyme disease in a particular way. Principles of naturopathic medicine inform everything I do and provide a foundation for the prevention and treatment strategies I review in this book.

Naturopathic physicians are educated and trained at 4-year naturopathic medical colleges that are accredited by the Council on Naturopathic Medical Education (CNME) and have passed professional

Reported Cases of Lyme Disease

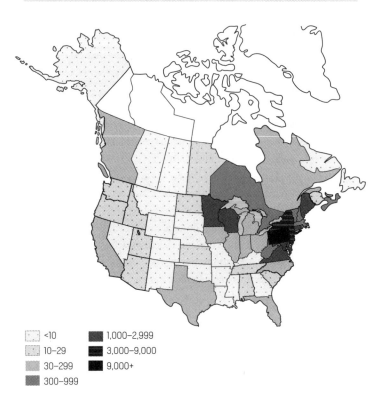

Legend:
- <10
- 10–29
- 30–299
- 300–999
- 1,000–2,999
- 3,000–9,000
- 9,000+

NOTE: The data shown here reflects reporting to the U.S. CDC in 2017 and the Public Health Agency of Canada in 2016. The state of Massachusetts monitors Lyme incidence differently than most states, and most of its confirmed cases are not reported to the CDC, so this map does not accurately represent that state.

board examinations administered by the North American Board of Naturopathic Examiners (NABNE) in order to become licensed. In addition to following a standard medical curriculum, a naturopathic doctor studies clinical nutrition, homeopathic medicine, botanical medicine, psychology, hydrotherapy, and counseling. Naturopathic medicine is based on the belief that the body has an innate ability to heal. Serving as both specialists and primary care physicians, naturopaths combine conventional diagnostics and treatment with natural therapies.

As of this writing, licensure of naturopathic physicians is state by state. I am licensed in Vermont; my scope of practice includes full prescription medication rights and ordering lab work, and I am covered by Vermont insurance.

The Father of Naturopathy

Dr. Benedict Lust (1872–1945) was the father of American naturopathy. Originally from Germany, he studied with many "nature-curists" in Europe. Having received his doctor of osteopathic medicine degree from the Universal Osteopathic College of New York and his doctor of medicine degree from the New York Homeopathic Medical College, he went on to open the first naturopathic college in America (American School of Naturopathy in New York).

Principles of Naturopathic Medicine

There are six principles of naturopathic medicine that provide the foundation to the unique philosophy held by naturopaths. The principles guide a naturopathic doctor's approach to interviewing a patient, critical thinking in creating differential diagnoses, medical decision-making, and collaborating with the patient.

1. **SUPPORT THE HEALING POWER OF NATURE.** Naturopathic medicine supports the inherent ability in each of us to heal.

2. **IDENTIFY AND TREAT THE CAUSE.** Investigation into the patient's complete health history is essential in discovering the cause of illness. Focus is placed on treating the cause, not just the symptoms.

3. **FIRST, DO NO HARM.** Noninvasive, nontoxic methods of diagnosis and treatment are used first.

4. **THE DOCTOR IS A TEACHER.** For a patient, understanding how the body works, its ability to heal, and medical diagnoses and treatment is an important part of the healing process.

5. **TREAT THE WHOLE PERSON.** Naturopathic medicine takes a holistic look at all of the physical body systems, as well as addressing mental, emotional, environmental, social, and spiritual health.

6. **PREVENTION IS THE BEST MEDICINE.** Assessing risk factors for disease and choosing a healthy lifestyle are the key to a longer, healthier life.

As you can see, naturopathic medicine takes a whole-person approach to healing acute and chronic illness. In particular, the principles above guide how I think about wellness and dis-ease in the body, and how I empower my patients through education and encourage them to trust in their body's innate wisdom. Finally, the last principle, prevention, has spurred me to learn about the preventive tools and strategies that are the focus of this book.

Roadmap

In this book, chapters 1 and 2 provide background on tick-borne diseases and ticks, the arachnids that carry and transmit these diseases. Chapter 3 describes where ticks thrive, how to decrease the tick population in your neck of the woods, and how to prevent tick bites. Chapter 4 explains how to prepare your body to be better equipped to handle a tick bite before it happens and if it happens. Chapter 5 discusses what to do if you get a tick bite, including tick removal and identification, homeopathic first aid, tick testing, immediate tick bite treatment, and symptoms to watch for. Chapter 6 explains what steps to take if you develop symptoms, what to do if you are diagnosed with acute Lyme or TBD, and how to find a Lyme-literate practitioner. The Resources section has detailed information about organizations that are referenced throughout the book, including useful services, trusted sources for herbs, educational organizations, and laboratories. These practical tools can empower each of us to help stop the spread of Lyme and tick-borne disease one person at a time.

Naturopathic medicine takes a whole-person approach to healing acute and chronic illness.

CHAPTER 1

Ticks

Ticks are biting arachnids that are widespread globally and are problematic due to the diseases they can transmit to humans. In this chapter, we'll review the most common ticks in North America, where they are located, and the pathogens they can carry. Most importantly, we will examine how best to identify ticks, which is key to determining the risk for various tick-borne diseases, like Lyme disease.

The distribution maps will tell you which ticks are found in your state or province. However, the maps do not reflect the nuances of tick population regionality within a state or province or whether those ticks are pathogenic (carrying pathogens that may be transmitted to you from a bite). For more specific information, connect with your local department of health or USDA Cooperative Extension Office to determine the pathogenicity of ticks in your state.

Species in North America

TICKS ARE PARASITIC ARACHNIDS: they depend on a host's blood for nutrition. An ixodid (hard) tick needs three blood meals in order to grow from a larva to a nymph to an adult. To find a blood meal, a tick will sense for body heat and carbon dioxide coming from a potential host and begin "questing." Questing is the act of a tick holding on to something in its environment — a blade of grass, a bit of leaf litter, the fibers of a dog bed — with its third and/or fourth pair of legs while reaching out with its first two pairs of legs, waiting to grab hold of a passerby.

Ticks exist worldwide. The ticks discussed in this chapter are found in North America. Most are ixodid (hard) ticks from the family Ixodidae. Each type of tick is restricted to or prevalent in a certain region and may carry specific pathogens — microorganisms capable of causing disease. I recommend becoming familiar with the type of ticks in your geographical area and those areas you may visit.

NOTE: The Tick ID card at the end of this book features full-color images of each of the ticks profiled over the following pages, at their actual size, which is helpful for identification purposes.

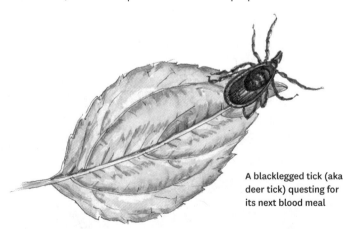

A blacklegged tick (aka deer tick) questing for its next blood meal

Blacklegged Tick (aka Deer Tick)

SPECIES: *Ixodes scapularis*

POSSIBLE PATHOGENS CARRIED: *Borrelia burgdorferi*, *B. mayonii*, *B. miyamotoi*, *Babesia* species, *Anaplasma phagocytophilum*, *Ehrlichia muris eauclairensis*, and Powassan virus

NOTE: While small numbers of blacklegged ticks, also known as deer ticks, have been shown to carry *Coxiella burnetii* and *Bartonella* species, these pathogens have not been shown to be transmitted from tick to human. In 2019, a study testing *Ixodes scapularis* in New York and Connecticut showed that 56.3 percent carried *Borrelia burgdorferi*, 10.6 percent carried *Anaplasma phagocytophilum*, 7.6 percent carried *Babesia microti*, 5 percent carried *Borrelia miyamotoi*, and 3.6 percent carried Powassan virus. In addition, the study reported that 16 percent were found to carry two pathogens and 3 percent were found to carry three pathogens. In fact, experts estimate that 2 to 10 percent of all ticks that transmit Lyme disease, via the *B. burdgdorferi* bacterium, also carry *B. miyamotoi*, a bacterium that causes tick-borne relapsing fever.[1]

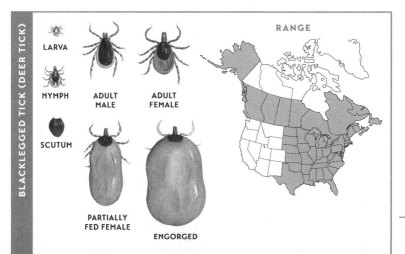

BLACKLEGGED TICK (DEER TICK)

LARVA

NYMPH

ADULT MALE

ADULT FEMALE

SCUTUM

PARTIALLY FED FEMALE

ENGORGED

RANGE

Western Blacklegged Tick
(aka Western Deer Tick)

SPECIES: *Ixodes pacificus*

POSSIBLE PATHOGENS CARRIED: *Borrelia burgdorferi*, *B. miyamotoi*, and *Anaplasma phagocytophilum*. It is most likely the vector that has transmitted *Babesia duncani* to people on the West Coast.[2]

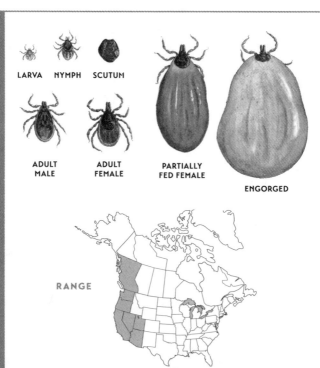

LARVA NYMPH SCUTUM

ADULT MALE

ADULT FEMALE

PARTIALLY FED FEMALE

ENGORGED

RANGE

American Dog Tick

SPECIES: *Dermacentor variabilis*

POSSIBLE PATHOGENS CARRIED: *Rickettsia rickettsii* and *Francisella tularensis*

NOTE: The dog tick is sometimes called the wood tick. Though it is often considered a primary vector of *R. rickettsii*, it has, in fact, been found to carry this pathogen infrequently.[3]

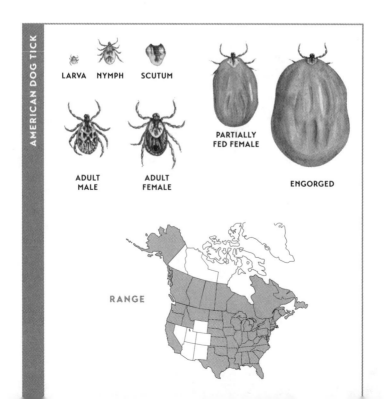

AMERICAN DOG TICK

LARVA   NYMPH   SCUTUM

PARTIALLY FED FEMALE

ADULT MALE   ADULT FEMALE

ENGORGED

RANGE

Lone Star Tick

SPECIES: *Amblyomma americanum*

POSSIBLE PATHOGENS CARRIED: *Ehrlichia chaffeensis*, *E. ewingii*, *Francisella tularensis*, and Heartland virus. While another pathogen, *Rickettsia amblyommatis*, has been found in lone star ticks, as of 2018 it had not been determined whether it causes disease.[4] Although recent comprehensive review of numerous studies has concluded that the lone star tick does not carry *Borrelia burgdorferi*,[5] the bacterium that causes Lyme disease, it has been found to carry *Borrelia lonestari*, the bacterium that is thought to be one possible cause of southern tick-associated rash illness (STARI).[6] I suspect that in the near future new data will definitively prove that lone star ticks carry *Borrelia* species.

NOTES: In comparison to deer ticks, lone star ticks move faster. Lone star larvae also stick together after hatching and can attach to their host in a cluster of hundreds.

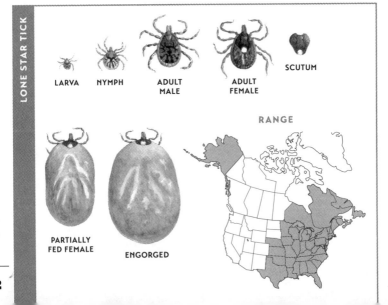

LONE STAR TICK

LARVA NYMPH ADULT MALE ADULT FEMALE SCUTUM

PARTIALLY FED FEMALE ENGORGED

RANGE

Alpha-Gal Syndrome

Lone star ticks carry the carbohydrate alpha-gal in their saliva. When a lone star tick bites a human, an allergic response can occur. Since humans do not make alpha-gal, but other nonprimate mammals do, our immune system can create anti-alpha-gal IgE antibodies when coming into contact with alpha-gal after eating mammalian meat like beef, pork, or lamb. The result is an allergic reaction called alpha-gal syndrome, which can happen up to 8 hours after exposure.

The symptoms of alpha-gal syndrome include the following after consuming beef, pork, or lamb:

× Hives or itching

× Itching or swelling in the mouth, lips, face, tongue, or throat; throat closing

× Runny nose or sneezing

× Abdominal pain, diarrhea, nausea, or vomiting

× Headaches

× Trouble breathing or anaphylaxis

Anyone with alpha-gal syndrome should avoid mammalian meat and sometimes also dairy products and certain medications. The allergy may resolve over time.

Interestingly, while anti-alpha-gal IgE antibodies are associated with tick-induced allergy (i.e., alpha-gal syndrome) in humans, anti-alpha-gal IgG/IgM antibodies may protect people against malaria, leishmaniasis, and Chagas disease.[7] I predict that more research will clarify alpha-gal's effect on the human immune system in relationship to infectious diseases. Anti-alpha-gal IgG/IgM antibodies may be tested for through bloodwork.

Brown Dog Tick

SPECIES: *Rhipicephalus sanguineus*

POSSIBLE PATHOGEN CARRIED:
Rickettsia rickettsii

NOTE: Brown dog ticks rarely transmit disease to humans. Dogs are the primary host and will receive pathogens from these ticks. Home or kennel infestations are possible since these ticks can live indoors for their entire lives.

RANGE

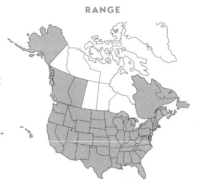

Gulf Coast Tick

SPECIES: *Amblyomma maculatum*

POSSIBLE PATHOGENS CARRIED:
Rickettsia parkeri and *Ehrlichia chaffeensis*

RANGE

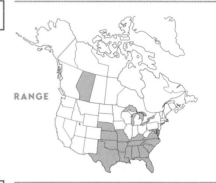

Rocky Mountain Wood Tick

SPECIES: *Dermacentor andersoni*

POSSIBLE PATHOGENS CARRIED:
Rickettsia rickettsii, Francisella tularensis, and the virus that causes Colorado tick fever

RANGE

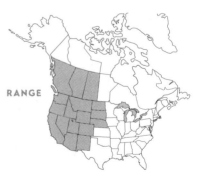

TICKS

BROWN DOG TICK

LARVA

NYMPH

ADULT
MALE

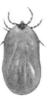

ADULT
FEMALE

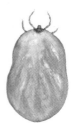

SCUTUM

PARTIALLY
FED FEMALE

ENGORGED

GULF COAST TICK

LARVA

NYMPH

ADULT
MALE

ADULT
FEMALE

SCUTUM

PARTIALLY
FED FEMALE

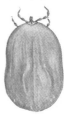

ENGORGED

ROCKY MOUNTAIN WOOD TICK

LARVA

NYMPH

ADULT
MALE

ADULT
FEMALE

SCUTUM

PARTIALLY
FED FEMALE

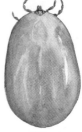

ENGORGED

Ornithodoros Tick

SPECIES: *Ornithodoros hermsi*, *O. parkeri*, and *O. turicata*

POSSIBLE PATHOGENS CARRIED: *Ornithodoros* tick species can carry *Borrelia* species, and those bacteria are named for the tick that carries them. *O. hermsi* can carry *Borrelia hermsii*, *O. parkeri* can carry *B. parkeri*, and *O. turicata* can carry *B. turicatae*. These three *Borrelia* species cause tick-borne relapsing fever.

NOTES: *Ornithodoros* is a member of the family of soft-bodied ticks called Argasidae. These are the only argasid (soft) ticks we will discuss in this book. These ticks have characteristics that are different from those of ixodid (hard) ticks: they do not have a dorsal shield (scutum), males and females look the same, their mouthparts are not visible from above, they feed rapidly, and humans are incidental hosts. *Ornithodoros* species live in rodent burrows and feed on those rodents at night.

    Ornithodoros hermsi are found at high altitudes, while *O. parkeri* are usually found at lower altitudes. *O. turicata* are also found at lower altitudes, including in caves.

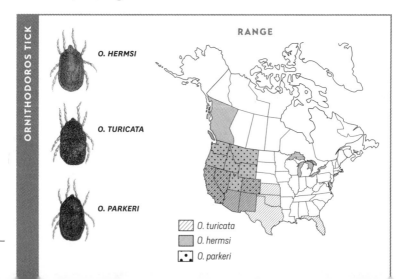

ORNITHODOROS TICK

RANGE

O. HERMSI

O. TURICATA

O. PARKERI

   O. turicata
   O. hermsi
   O. parkeri

Asian Longhorned Tick

SPECIES: *Haemaphysalis longicornis*

POSSIBLE PATHOGENS CARRIED: As of this writing, the Asian long-horned tick has not been found to carry pathogens that cause illness in animals or humans in the United States.[9] Curiously, though, it does carry and transmit diseases in its native eastern Asia. Ongoing research in the United States is necessary to identify any emerging pathogens in this tick.

NOTE: The Asian longhorned tick was found in North America for the first time in 2017, in New Jersey; since that time it has spread quickly, with its range as of August 2019 shown in the map below. Female Asian longhorned ticks can reproduce without mating, which contributes to their ability to spread quickly. If you find an Asian long-horned tick, contact your local department of health.

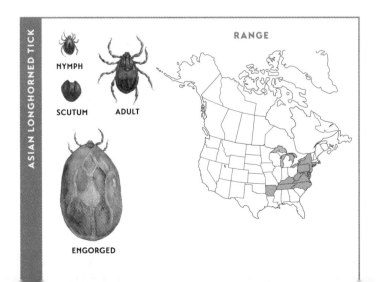

ASIAN LONGHORNED TICK

NYMPH

SCUTUM   ADULT

ENGORGED

RANGE

Tick Identification

THE BEST WAY TO IDENTIFY a hard-bodied tick is by examining its dorsal shield, or scutum, a hard (sclerotized) plate on its back. The deer ticks *Ixodes scapularis* and *I. pacificus* have a solid black-brown scutum, whereas *Dermacentor variabilis* (American dog or wood tick) has a mottled brown-and-white scutum. Adult female lone star ticks are easy to identify by a single white dot on their brown scutum, in the middle of their body. A tick's dorsal shield looks the same at each stage of life, and it will stay the same size and color regardless of how bloated the tick may become after a blood meal. See the Tick ID guide at the end of this book for a close-up look at the dorsal shield of each species.

Ixodes scapularis (deer ticks) are also smaller than the *Dermacentor variabilis* (American dog or wood ticks). An adult female deer tick is half the size of an American dog tick. An adult female deer tick is the size of a sesame seed (2.5 mm), whereas a nymph is the size of a poppy seed (1 mm). Larvae are the size of the period at the end of this sentence (0.5 mm). For a look at the actual size of the various tick species, again, see the Tick ID guide at the end of this book.

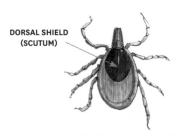

DORSAL SHIELD (SCUTUM)

Mature blacklegged (deer) tick

The Tick Life Cycle

UNDERSTANDING THE IXODID (hard) tick life cycle can help you know what to watch for during tick season. An *Ixodes scapularis* tick emerges from an egg mass as a larva in summer. The larva will attach to a small animal, like a white-footed mouse. If the mouse is carrying a pathogen, such as *Borrelia burgdorferi*, which causes Lyme disease, the tick larva may acquire the pathogen through the blood meal. After its first blood meal, the larva will drop off its host, develop another pair of legs, grow in size, and become a nymph. The nymph overwinters, usually under leaf litter or vegetation (or snow). In springtime, the nymph moves to low-growing vegetation and waits for a new host — anything from a mouse or bird to a dog or human. The nymph will attach to its new host and take its next blood meal, during which time it may acquire and/or transmit pathogens to/from its host. Once engorged, the nymph drops off its host into grass, leaf litter, a dog bed, your couch — wherever it is. It molts into an adult. In fall, the adult tick will attach to a larger animal such as a dog, deer, or human, and now, too, it may transmit pathogens it is carrying to the host. It will again overwinter, and the female will lay eggs in spring. The life cycle of *Ixodes pacificus* is the same as that of *I. scapularis* except that it is shifted a bit later: larvae and nymphs become active in late spring until summer, while adults are active from late fall through spring.

At this time, the only known pathogen transmitted by deer tick larvae is *Borrelia miyamotoi*, which causes tick-borne relapsing fever. It is the only *Borrelia* species known to be transmitted

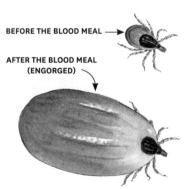

BEFORE THE BLOOD MEAL →

AFTER THE BLOOD MEAL
(ENGORGED) ↘

During a blood meal, an adult deer tick can expand to up to 200 times its original size.

The Tick Life Cycle

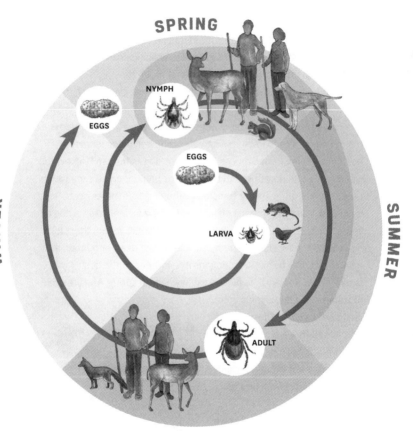

SPRING

NYMPH

EGGS

EGGS

WINTER

LARVA

SUMMER

ADULT

FALL

from the adult tick to the larvae. For all other tick-borne diseases, ticks acquire the pathogens from their first blood meal as larvae or from their second blood meal as nymphs. Nymphs and adults are the life stages that transmit all other tick-borne disease.

An adult male will feed a small amount in order to mate, while an adult female needs a full blood meal to lay eggs. An unmated female deer tick (*Ixodes scapularis* and *I. pacificus*) will feed enough to increase to 10 times its original size. A mated female deer tick will expand to 100 to 200 times its original size. The adult female will then lay an egg mass, containing up to 3,000 eggs, in spring that will hatch in summer to repeat the same 2-year cycle.

Note, however, that the above-described tick life cycle does not apply to argasid (soft) ticks, such as the *Ornithodoros* genus. Instead, *Ornithodoros* ticks live for many years and therefore have two or more nymphal stages, each of which requires a blood meal.

Tick Education:
A Resource for Teachers

Global Lyme Alliance (GLA) has created free curriculum and teacher workbooks about ticks and Lyme disease for grades K through 12. Visit the website at GLA.org to download and print the workbooks or use the digital interactive version of the workbooks. Students will learn about ticks, Lyme disease, and tick bite prevention through this interactive curriculum and earn a "Lyme Alert" certificate upon completion. This curriculum is appropriate for places like school and camp.

It is essential to equip the next generation with the information they need to prevent tick bites and tick-borne disease. The GLA curriculum, in particular, will especially impact the age group of five- to nine-year-olds, who comprise the demographic for the highest number of new Lyme disease cases.

CHAPTER 2

Lyme and Tick-Borne Disease

Lyme disease is the most commonly diagnosed and most familiar tick-borne disease. In addition to Lyme disease, ticks carry other pathogens that may be bacteria, protozoa, or viruses that can cause other diseases. In this chapter, we'll discuss in detail the top tick-borne diseases diagnosed in North America. We will review each organism causing each disease and the time it takes to develop symptoms, as well as the symptoms caused by each disease.

Reading the Maps

The discussion of each disease is accompanied by a map showing the areas in the US and Canada where it has been reported. There are a few things to keep in mind about these maps:

×   In general, tick-borne diseases are widely underreported across the United States and Canada. The maps show only *reported* cases. A disease that has not been reported in a particular area may, nevertheless, be present in that area.

×   The states and provinces that are highlighted in the maps show where tick-borne disease has been reported, and not necessarily where it was contracted.

×   If a disease is said to be "not notifiable" for a particular state or province, that means that the state or province does not require medical practitioners to report cases of that disease, and so we lack statistics about the incidence of that disease.

×   There can be tremendous variability in the incidence of tick-borne disease within states and provinces. A tick or tick-borne disease that is present in one part of a state may not be present in other parts of that state.

×   To find out which tick-borne diseases are present in your state or province, consult the chart on pages 172–173. For more accurate information about which diseases are present in your specific region of your state or province, contact your local department of health.

Snapshot: Tick-Borne Disease in the United States

DISEASE	TIME PERIOD	NUMBER OF REPORTED CASES
Lyme disease	2017	42,743
Anaplasmosis	2017	5,762
Babesiosis	2015	2,074
Ehrlichiosis	2017	1,642+
Rickettsiosis*	2017	6,248
Tularemia	2017	239
Powassan virus	2009–2018	144
Heartland virus	Total as of Sept. 2018	40+
Tick-borne relapsing fever	1990–2011	483
Colorado tick fever	2002–2012	83
STARI	Unknown	Unknown
Q fever†	2017	193
Bartonellosis†	2005–2013	12,000 per year[9]

NOTE: Many of these diseases are present in Canada but not reportable, so we lack statistics to cite. What we do know is that in 2017, there were 2,025 cases of Lyme disease reported to the Canadian government.

*This figure includes *Rickettsia rickettsii*, *R. parkeri*, Pacific coast tick fever, and rickettsial pox (which is mite-borne) due to the inability to differentiate between spotted fever group *Rickettsia* species using serologic testing.

†I include Q fever and bartonellosis in this chart because experts suspect that these diseases may be transmitted by ticks, but please note that at the moment there is no definitive evidence to support this hypothesis.

Lyme Disease

LYME DISEASE IS A PREVENTABLE INFECTIOUS DISEASE that is transmitted through a tick bite, although fewer than half of people with Lyme disease actually recall a tick bite. Lyme disease, or Lyme borreliosis, is caused by a bacterium that has existed for millions of years. Lyme disease was discovered in Lyme, Connecticut, in 1975 by Dr. Alan Steere after a high number of children were diagnosed with what was thought to be juvenile rheumatoid arthritis. The bacterium itself was discovered in 1982 by entomologist Willy Burgdorfer and so was appropriately named *Borrelia burgdorferi*.

The term *Borrelia burgdorferi* is used in two different ways. There is the broad term *Borrelia burgdorferi* sensu lato (*sensu lato* means "in the broad sense"), which at the time of this writing includes 19 species of *Borrelia*. The more specific term *B. burgdorferi* sensu stricto (*sensu stricto* means "in the narrow sense") refers specifically to the *B. burgdorferi* species. Of the 19 species in the sensu lato classification, four (to date) have been proven to cause Lyme disease: *B. burgdorferi, B. mayonii, B. afzelii,* and *B. garinii.* (*Borrelia afzelii* and *B. garinii* are currently found only in Europe but may

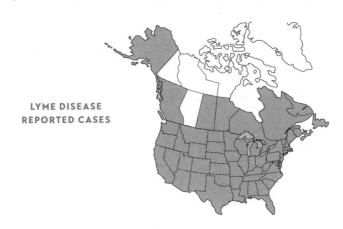

LYME DISEASE REPORTED CASES

arrive on this continent someday.) More *Borrelia* species are being discovered often.

Traditionally, bacteria can be categorized according to whether they are gram-positive or gram-negative — that is, whether they hold a stain (Gram's stain) in laboratory testing, which tells us about the structure of their cell wall. *Borrelia* is an atypical bacterium; it is neither gram-positive nor gram-negative. It is classified as a spirochete, meaning that is is helically shaped, like a corkscrew. Spirochetes are unique among bacteria for their arrangement of flagella (filament-like structures), which extend out through their cell membrane in a manner that allows them to move by rotating. The flagella give *Borrelia* excellent motility — which is especially helpful for moving through tissues in an infected host.

The relationship between *Borrelia* and a tick is symbiotic — both benefit. Ticks infected with *Borrelia* are more hydrated, which allows them to move more quickly, have longer life spans, take larger blood meals, and have larger fat stores. For its part, *Borrelia* requires a host to reproduce and does so through binary fission every 12 to 24 hours. It does not have the ability to make nucleotides, amino acids, fatty acids, or enzyme cofactors and therefore must live within a host to acquire those nutrients to survive.

The *Borrelia* bacterium has the unique ability to express a wide variety of lipoproteins on the surface of its outer membrane. These lipoproteins, or outer membrane surface proteins (Osp), express changes depending on where the bacterium is in the tick, whether the tick is attached to a host, whether the bacterium is transferred into a mammalian host, and what sort of response the mammalian host's immune system has to the bacterium. Variability in these outer membrane surface proteins allows for more effective invasion of the host.

Inside the unfed tick, *Borrelia* lives in the midgut and its surface proteins express as what is known as type A (OspA). OspA has unique structures that allow the bacterium to survive in the tick's midgut and bind to a receptor in the midgut lining that, for now, is generically known as TROSPA (tick receptor OspA).

When the tick attaches to a host and begins to feed, the temperature and pH in its midgut begin to change. These changes trigger *Borrelia*'s surface proteins to switch their expression from type A to type C. OspC does not bind to the tick's midgut. Now the bacterium is released, begins to multiply, and moves into the tick's salivary glands.

In the salivary glands, *Borrelia* biochemically analyzes the environment of the mammal host through the incoming blood meal and alters its genetic structure in order to prepare it for the new environment of its imminent host. A protein from the tick's saliva (Salp15) binds to the OspC on the bacterium. Salp15 aids the bacterium's transition from the tick to the mammalian host.

OspC protects the bacterium from the host's immune response, which is to make antibodies to the bacterium. Salp15 interferes with the host immune system in various ways, including intervening in the host's initial immune response to a pathogen like *Borrelia*. *Borrelia burgdorferi* itself has the ability to express many other surface proteins that can interact with the host immune system in order to resist annihilation.

Once *B. burgdorferi* is inside a mammal host, the host's immune system interacts with the bacterium's outer membrane surface proteins, which promptly rearrange themselves to help the bacterium resist annihilation. (As one set of researchers said, these surface proteins are "peerless immune evasion tools.")[10] With the immune system held in check, the bacterium moves through the host's tissues, collecting nutrients along the way. It populates capillaries and veins, and its surface proteins bind with human proteins involved in wound healing and blood clotting, assembly of connective tissue, production of cartilage, and communication between cell membranes and the extracellular matrix.[11] *Borrelia* penetrates connective tissue and invades synovial, neuronal, and glial cells. (Synovial cells line the joints and secrete synovial fluid that lubricates the joint cartilage; cartilage creates collagen, a protein that serves as food for the *Borrelia* bacterium. Neuronal cells are brain cells, while glial cells function as the connective tissue of the brain.) In this way, *B. burgdorferi* can invade the joints, brain, and heart, with wide-reaching effects on human health.

In the human body, *B. burgdorferi* is persistent and resilient in part due to the way the bacterium can change from the spirochete form to other forms. To begin, blebs — small, saclike outgrowths containing DNA and surface proteins — may protrude through the cell wall of the spirochete, eventually separating and floating free. Those blebs may become round body forms (also called cell wall–deficient forms). The typical response of the human immune system to invasion by pathogenic bacteria is to release macrophages (a type of white blood cell) that engulf the bacteria and destroy them. However, macrophages recognize and destroy round bodies less readily than they do spirochetes. Round bodies also initiate a different cytokine response from the immune system than do spirochetes. Cytokines are proteins secreted by certain cells of the immune system that regulate various inflammatory responses. The cytokine response to *B. burgdorferi* in its round body form has been shown to contribute to the development of Lyme arthritis.[12] Interestingly, research has also shown that *B. burgdorferi*

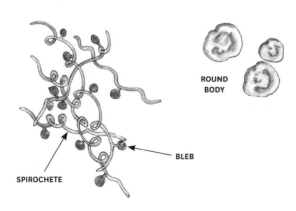

ROUND
BODY

BLEB

SPIROCHETE

spirochetes can be triggered to take on the round body form when they come into contact with antibiotics.

In another useful (for the bacteria) strategy, a community of *B. burgdorferi* spirochetes can come together in the human body and create a structure around themselves called biofilm. Think of biofilm as a slimy mass (made of mucoid polysaccharides and proteins) that surrounds the *Borrelia* community and allows it to hide from the human immune system and antibiotics. Researcher Eva Sapi describes it as a city of sorts.[13] Within this "city" may be numerous other types of microorganisms in addition to *B. burgdorferi*, all communicating, storing energy, transferring genetic information, and disposing of waste. Biofilm protects the organisms from the high temperatures and changes in pH to which they are vulnerable within the human host. When the city grows to a certain size, it splits into and releases smaller biofilm communities, in this manner spreading through and colonizing the host.

Borrelia burgdorferi also has an unusual genome that may contribute to its ability to persist in a host: it contains one linear chromosome and 21 plasmids, the highest number of plasmids of any bacterium. Plasmids are pieces of genetic information stored separately from a chromosome that can be shared with other bacteria during the reproductive process. They encode the outer surface proteins expressed by *Borrelia*. Thanks in part to these plasmids, there are many strains of *Borrelia burgdorferi* — that is, subspecies with slight genetic variation. Plasmids also play a major role in the overall infectivity of *Borrelia*.

After a bite from a tick carrying *Borrelia burgdorferi*, a human can develop borreliosis, better known as Lyme disease. A decrease in white blood cells (leukopenia) or an increase in white blood cells (leukocytosis), a decrease in platelets (thrombocytopenia), elevated liver enzymes, elevated sedimentation rate, and elevated creatine phosphokinase may be seen in the blood of a human with Lyme disease.

The Stages of Biofilm Development

Biofilm protects *Borrelia burgdorferi* and other microorganisms from the body's immune system.

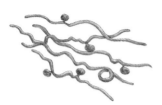 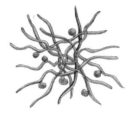

EARLY STAGES: Microorganisms such as *Borrelia* spirochetes begin to clump together and produce mucoid polysaccharides and proteins.

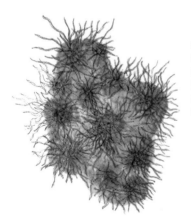

FULLY FORMED: The slimy mass of biofilm pervades and encapsulates the microbial community, protecting it from the body's immune system and facilitating exchanges between the resident microorganisms.

SPLITTING: Eventually the biofilm community splits, forming new, smaller communities that can spread in the body.

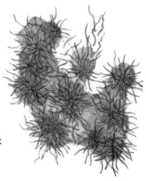

Signs and Symptoms of Lyme Disease

× Rash (erythema migrans): A pink or red rash surrounding the tick bite that:

- May or may not feel warm to the touch
- May or may not be circular with central clearing (that makes it look like a bull's-eye)
- May be flat or raised
- Usually spreads in a centrifugal fashion from around the bite outward
- May manifest as multiple rashes across the body (known as disseminated erythema migrans)

× Flu-like symptoms (fever and chills, unusual fatigue, headache)

× Swollen lymph nodes

× Joint pain and/or swelling

× Muscle pain

× Fatigue

× Headache

× Stiff neck

× Heart symptoms: chest pain, shortness of breath, palpitations, fainting

× Eye symptoms: redness of eyes, itchy or burning eyes, discharge, floaters

× Neurological symptoms: Bell's palsy or facial nerve (cranial nerve VII) palsy (the drooping of one or both sides of the face due to loss of muscle control), numbness, tingling, burning, shooting pain, weakness, cognitive changes, memory loss, mood changes, personality changes, seizures, confusion, pain with eye movement, double vision, ringing in ears, hearing loss, vertigo, problems walking, difficulty with balance

NOTE: The bull's-eye rash is perhaps the most well-known symptom of Lyme disease, but fewer than half of patients recall ever having a bull's-eye rash. The erythema migrans can manifest in many other patterns, too, including those listed at left. See the photos on the identification guide at the end of this book for a look at some of these alternative presentations of erythema migrans.

Symptoms of Lyme disease usually occur between 3 and 30 days after a tick bite but can take months to appear. Proper comprehensive early treatment usually results in full recovery. See chapter 6 for recommendations regarding early comprehensive treatment.

Persistent symptoms from a *Borrelia burgdorferi* infection can occur after contraction of Lyme disease, even after antibiotic treatment. The spirochete's survival mechanism, which allows it to change forms and to hide in biofilm, and its expression of surface proteins can help it evade the immune system, while it may also release proteins that inactivate certain immune system responses. *B. burgdorferi*'s outer surface proteins may also mimic human cells, so that a person's immune system accidentally attacks itself in addition to the invading bacteria.[14] Additionally, there may be other *Borrelia* species that have not been killed by antibiotics or other untreated tick-borne diseases that make it difficult for a person's immune system to resolve the infections. Eating a proinflammatory diet of foods like sugar, yeast, alcohol, grains, and processed foods may contribute to a lingering infection.

...

Lyme disease is the most common tick-borne disease in the United States, but many other pathogens carried by ticks in the United States may be transmitted to humans: anaplasmosis, babesiosis, ehrlichiosis, rickettsial spotted fever group, tularemia, Powassan virus, Heartland virus, tick-borne relapsing fever, Colorado tick fever, southern tick-associated rash illness, and possibly bartonellosis. We'll look at all these next.

Anaplasmosis

Anaplasmosis, another disease borne by deer ticks, is caused by the *Anaplasma phagocytophilum* bacterium. Anaplasmosis is also called human granulocytic anaplasmosis (HGA) and was previously called human granulocytic ehrlichiosis (HGE). *Anaplasma* is a gram-negative bacterium that infects neutrophils, a type of white blood cell, inside the host. A decrease in white blood cells (leukopenia), a decrease in platelets (thrombocytopenia), and elevated liver enzymes may be seen in the blood of a human with anaplasmosis.

Signs and Symptoms of Anaplasmosis

× Fever

× Severe headache

× Muscle pain

× Fatigue

× Nausea, vomiting, abdominal pain, loss of appetite

× Cough

× Rash: pinpoint or splotchy rash, typically not itchy, and sparing the face, palms, and soles

Symptoms occur between 5 and 21 days after a tick bite. Treatment usually results in full recovery.

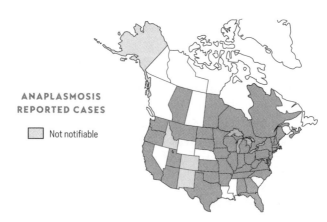

ANAPLASMOSIS
REPORTED CASES

Not notifiable

Babesiosis

Babesiosis is a deer tick–borne disease caused by *Babesia microti*, *B. divergens*, and *B. duncani*. The *Babesia* protozoan is malaria-like, reproducing in the red blood cells of the host. A decrease in red blood cells (hemolytic anemia), a decrease in platelets (thrombocytopenia), elevated creatinine and blood urea nitrogen (BUN), and elevated liver enzymes may be seen in the blood of a human with babesiosis.

Signs and Symptoms of Babesiosis

Some symptoms caused by babesiosis are similar to those caused by Lyme disease:

- Fever
- Chills
- Fatigue
- Headaches

- Muscle pain
- Joint pain

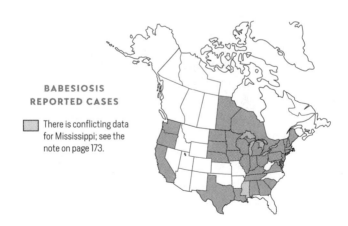

BABESIOSIS REPORTED CASES

There is conflicting data for Mississippi; see the note on page 173.

A classic babesiosis presentation includes:

- × Excessive sweating
- × Heart palpitations
- × Unexplained cough
- × "Air hunger" (difficulty breathing, even without exertion)
- × Chest pain

Symptoms can appear within 1 week or after several months from the tick bite. Babesiosis can be life threatening to people who do not have a spleen, the elderly, those with liver or kidney disease, and individuals whose immune system has been compromised.

Babesia Life Cycle

The deer tick first becomes infected with *Babesia* protozoans from a small animal when the tick attaches and receives gametocytes from the blood meal. (A gametocyte is a reproductive cell passed from a host to the tick.) When the tick transmits *Babesia* to a larger animal like a human, it enters the animal's red blood cells in a form called sporozoites. In the red blood cells, they multiply by way of binary fission. Sporozoites become trophozoites, which then become merozoites. The trophozoites and merozoites together make up vermicules, which are packages of *Babesia*. The vermicules rupture the red blood cell and therefore release *Babesia* into the bloodstream.

Ehrlichiosis

Ehrlichiosis is caused by bacteria transmitted typically by lone star and Gulf coast ticks. It is also called human monocytotropic ehrlichiosis (HME) and is caused by *Ehrlichia chaffeensis*, *E. ewingii*, or *E. muris eauclairensis* (formerly called *Ehrlichia muris*–like agent). *Ehrlichia* is a gram-negative bacterium that infects monocytes, a type of white blood cell inside the host. Only 68 percent of people diagnosed with ehrlichiosis remember a tick bite.[15] There is a 3 percent fatality rate for *E. chaffeensis*, which causes more severe illness than *E. ewingii* or *E. muris eauclairensis*. A decrease in white blood cells (leukopenia), a decrease in platelets (thrombocytopenia), and elevated liver enzymes may be seen in the blood of a human with ehrlichiosis. In 2011, *E. muris eauclairensis* was discovered in Wisconsin and Minnesota. The new species has been detected in the blacklegged tick, *Ixodes scapularis*, in Wisconsin and Minnesota.[16]

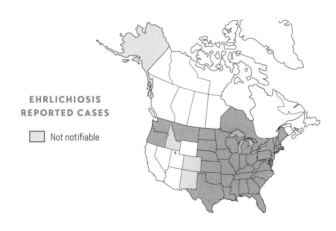

**EHRLICHIOSIS
REPORTED CASES**

Not notifiable

Signs and Symptoms of Ehrlichiosis

- × Fever
- × Headache
- × Muscle pain
- × Fatigue
- × Nausea, vomiting, abdominal pain, loss of appetite
- × Cough
- × Confusion
- × Rash: pinpoint or splotchy rash, typically not itchy and sparing the face, palms, and soles

Symptoms occur between 5 and 14 days after a tick bite. Treatment usually results in full recovery.

Rickettsial Spotted Fever Group

Spotted fever is a disease caused by an infection with rickettsial bacteria. *Rickettsia* is a genus of gram-negative bacteria with a parasitic nature. There are more than 30 species and subspecies.[17] *Rickettsia* infects ticks as well as other arthropods worldwide. For our purposes, we will focus on the rickettsial spotted fever group, which infects ticks in North America. Rocky Mountain spotted fever (RMSF) is caused by *Rickettsia rickettsii*, which is carried by the American dog, brown dog, and Rocky Mountain wood ticks. Other spotted fever group (SFG) rickettsial disease is caused by *Rickettsia parkeri*, which is carried by the Gulf coast tick, and *R. philipii*, which is carried by the *Dermacentor occidentalis* tick (see page 51).

Rickettsia invades the endothelial cells of blood vessels in humans. When capillaries are broken by the bacteria, the result is the hallmark appearance of Rocky Mountain spotted fever — petechiae, a red or purple spotted rash. Less than 50 percent of people have the rash within the first 3 days of illness, and a smaller percentage never develop a rash. Children are more likely to develop the rash. Only 55 to 60 percent of people who were diagnosed with Rocky Mountain spotted fever[18] remember having a tick bite. There is a fatality rate of 5 to 10 percent for those who contract Rocky Mountain spotted fever. Fatality rates are disproportionately higher in young children. A slight increase in white blood cells (leukocytosis), decrease in platelets (thrombocytopenia), slightly elevated liver enzymes, and low sodium (hyponatremia) may be seen in the blood of a human with Rocky Mountain spotted fever, with similar but milder findings in people with *Rickettsia parkeri* rickettsiosis.

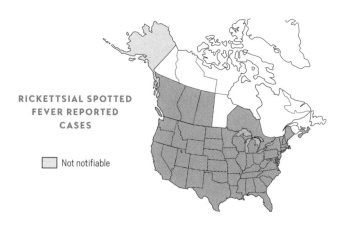

RICKETTSIAL SPOTTED FEVER REPORTED CASES

Not notifiable

Signs and Symptoms of Rocky Mountain Spotted Fever (*R. rickettsii* Infection):

Days 1–4

- Fever
- Headache
- Chills
- Malaise
- Muscle pain
- Nausea, vomiting, abdominal pain, loss of appetite
- Light sensitivity
- Swelling around eyes and back of hands
- Rash: typically occurs 2 to 4 days after onset of fever, starting with a flat, pink rash on the ankles, wrists, or forearms and spreading to the palms, soles, arms, legs, and trunk, usually sparing the face; it may create petechiae (clusters of tiny, flat, circular spots on the surface of the skin caused by bleeding under the skin) and may become a raised pink, red, or purple rash

Days 5+

- Confusion, changes in mental state
- Difficulty breathing

Symptoms of Rocky Mountain spotted fever occur between 3 and 12 days after a tick bite.

Signs and Symptoms of *R. parkeri* Rickettsiosis

- Eschar — a dry, dark scab or dead skin over an ulcer that may be surrounded by redness at the site of the tick bite; usually the first sign
- Fever
- Headache
- Muscle pain
- Lymph node swelling

- × Rash: typically occurs within 4 days after onset of fever; a flat or raised pink or red rash on the trunk, arms, legs, palms, soles, and face

Symptoms of *R. parkeri* rickettsiosis occur between 2 and 10 days after a tick bite.

Signs and Symptoms of *R. philipii* Rickettsiosis

- × Eschar or ulcer at the site of the tick bite
- × Fever
- × Headache
- × Muscle pain
- × Fatigue

R. philipii rickettsiosis is a newer, less common disease, and information on when its symptoms manifest is unavailable at the time of this writing. Research is ongoing.

Emerging Research: Pacific Coast Tick Watch

As of 2016, California had recorded 14 confirmed cases of Pacific coast tick fever, a disease caused by *R. philipii* that can be transmitted by a Pacific coast tick (*Dermacentor occidentalis*) bite.[19] Be on the lookout for more information regarding this tick and tick-borne disease in the future.

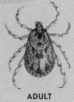

ADULT MALE   ADULT FEMALE

Tularemia

Tularemia, or rabbit fever, is a disease caused by *Francisella tularensis*. It is transmitted by the American dog, lone star, and Rocky Mountain wood ticks. It is a gram-negative bacterium that infects macrophages, a type of white blood cell. In addition to tick bites, tularemia is also spread through deerfly bites and contact with infected animals, such as rabbits, rodents, and sometimes birds, cats, and dogs.

Signs and Symptoms of Tick-Transmitted Tularemia

- ✕ Ulcer at the site of the tick bite
- ✕ Lymph node swelling, usually in the armpit or groin
- ✕ Fever
- ✕ Headache
- ✕ Chills

- ✕ Fatigue
- ✕ Sore throat
- ✕ Runny nose
- ✕ Nausea, vomiting, diarrhea
- ✕ If untreated, later symptoms may include cough, chest pain and difficulty breathing

Symptoms of tularemia occur between 3 and 15 days after a tick bite.

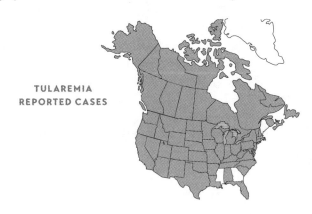

TULAREMIA REPORTED CASES

Powassan Virus

Powassan virus is the "only North American member of the tick-borne encephalitis serogroup of flaviviruses."[20] The transmission of the Powassan RNA virus from a tick to a host can happen very quickly, in as little as 15 minutes! While only found in less than 4 percent of *Ixodes scapularis* ticks, Powassan virus is fatal in 10 percent of cases. Fifty percent of people who develop neurological symptoms continue to experience long-lasting symptoms.

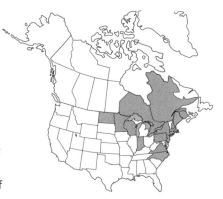

POWASSAN VIRUS REPORTED CASES

Signs and Symptoms of Powassan Virus

Early symptoms during the first week:

✗	Sore throat	✗	Headache
✗	Drowsiness	✗	Disorientation

Next phase, lasting weeks to months:

✗	Fever	✗	Loss of coordination
✗	Vomiting	✗	Seizures
✗	Difficulty breathing	✗	Lethargy
✗	Difficulty speaking	✗	Paralysis

Potential long-lasting symptoms:

✗	Memory problems	✗	Severe headaches
✗	Muscle wasting	✗	Paralysis

Symptoms of Powassan virus occur between 1 and 5 weeks after a tick bite.

Heartland Virus

Heartland virus, transmitted by the lone star tick, is caused by a virus (specifically, a member of the *Phlebovirus* genus). A decrease in white blood cells (leukopenia), a decrease in platelets (thrombocytopenia), and elevated liver enzymes may be seen in the blood of a human with Heartland virus. This is a recently discovered tick-borne RNA virus; 40 cases were reported nationwide as of September 2018.

Signs and Symptoms of Heartland Virus

- × Fever
- × Fatigue
- × Loss of appetite
- × Headache
- × Nausea
- × Diarrhea
- × Muscle pain
- × Joint pain

The incubation period is unknown, although most people with Heartland virus reported a tick bite within 2 weeks of illness onset.

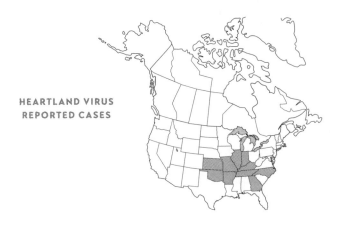

HEARTLAND VIRUS
REPORTED CASES

Tick-Borne Relapsing Fever

Although *Borrelia burgdorferi*, which causes Lyme disease, is the most studied organism, it is important to note that there are other species of *Borrelia* that cause other kinds of illness. There are 15 *Borrelia* species that cause tick-borne relapsing fever (TBRF) worldwide. *B. miyamotoi* is the only *Borrelia* species carried by an *Ixodes* (hard) tick that causes tick-borne relapsing fever. *B. miyamotoi* may be transmitted from the adult female *Ixodes* tick to its eggs, which results in infected tick larvae. All other TBRF *Borrelia* are transmitted from *Ornithodoros* (soft) ticks.

Most common in Africa, Central Asia, the Mediterranean, and Central and South America, cases of TBRF have been also been reported in western United States and Canada.[21] *Borrelia hermsii*, *B. parkeri*, and *B. turicatae* are the three species transmitted by *Ornithodoros* ticks that cause TBRF in the United States. Most commonly, a human may become infected after sleeping or working in a rodent-infested cabin, hunting camp, barn, or building. During the night, the tick may incidentally attach to a human for a short time and cause a painless bite. In the United States, TBRF occurs most

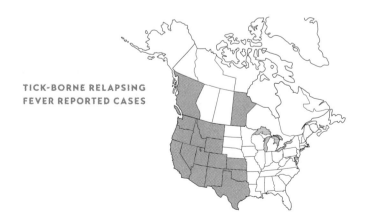

TICK-BORNE RELAPSING FEVER REPORTED CASES

commonly in 14 western states: Arizona, California, Colorado, Idaho, Kansas, Montana, Nevada, New Mexico, Oklahoma, Oregon, Texas, Utah, Washington, and Wyoming.[22]

TBRF may cause relapsing symptoms lasting 3 days, followed by 7 days without a fever, followed by another 3 days with a fever. Elevated liver enzymes may be seen in the blood of a human with TBRF.

Signs and Symptoms of Tick-Borne Relapsing Fever

Common symptoms:

- High fever
- Headache
- Muscle and joint pain
- Chills
- Sweats
- Nausea
- Vomiting

Less common symptoms:

- Rash
- Loss of appetite
- Stiff neck
- Cough
- Abdominal pain
- Confusion
- Light sensitivity or eye problems
- Tingling and numbness in extremities
- Facial nerve palsy
- Hearing loss

Symptoms begin 7 days after a tick bite. TBRF may resolve on its own after several months. However, given the complicated nature of *Borrelia* species and the diseases they cause, I'd recommend treating as described in chapter 6.

Colorado Tick Fever

Colorado tick fever, a disease borne by Rocky Mountain wood ticks, is caused by a virus (specifically, a member of the *Coltivirus* genus). It infects red blood cells. A decrease in white blood cells (leukopenia), a decrease in platelets (thrombocytopenia), and elevated lymphocytes (lymphocytosis) may be seen in the blood of a human with Colorado tick fever. Eighty-three cases of this RNA virus were reported from 2002 to 2012.

Signs and Symptoms of Colorado Tick Fever

- × Fever
- × Biphasic fever: fever for several days, followed by feeling well for several days, then a return of a fever for several days
- × Chills

- × Headache
- × Muscle pain
- × Fatigue
- × Sore throat
- × Abdominal pain
- × Vomiting
- × Rash

Symptoms of Colorado tick fever occur between 1 and 14 days after a tick bite.

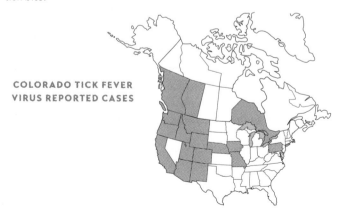

COLORADO TICK FEVER
VIRUS REPORTED CASES

Southern Tick-Associated Rash Illness

Southern tick-associated rash illness (STARI), or Masters disease, is a syndrome with unknown causes. Spirochetes that look similar to *Borrelia* were found in lone star ticks. Studies point to a connection between the pathogen, a lone star tick bite, and an illness that developed. At this time, there is not enough evidence to show a causal relationship between *Borrelia lonestari* and the illness people have exhibited called STARI after a lone star tick bite. However, I highly suspect that the bull's-eye-like rash seen in STARI is caused by a *Borrelia* species, since an erythema migrans is a classic proven manifestation of *B. burgdorferi* sensu stricto, the bacterium that causes Lyme disease. Furthermore, other symptoms that may be experienced by someone diagnosed with STARI mimic those of Lyme disease.

Signs and Symptoms of STARI

- ✗ Rash: similar to the Lyme rash
- ✗ Fever
- ✗ Flu-like symptoms
- ✗ Headaches
- ✗ Stiff neck
- ✗ Joint pain
- ✗ Muscle pain
- ✗ Fatigue

More research is imperative to learn about STARI and its cause. As of this writing, there is no surveillance of the disease, and therefore we do not know how many people have been infected. I suspect there may be a silent epidemic of STARI waiting to be uncovered.

NOTE: Distribution information on STARI is currently unavailable.

Bartonellosis

Bartonellosis is a disease caused by *Bartonella* species, which are gram-negative bacteria. They infect endothelial cells of blood vessels and multiply inside red blood cells. The disease exists worldwide. *Bartonella* species are most commonly transmitted to humans through contact with fleas and lice. For example, *B. henselae*, which causes cat scratch fever, is transmitted to humans via flea feces carried in cats' nails. Ticks can also carry *Bartonella* species. One study in New Jersey and another in California showed that some *Ixodes scapularis* and *I. pacificus* ticks, respectively, carried *Bartonella*.[23] However, no current evidence shows that ticks can transmit *Bartonella* to humans.

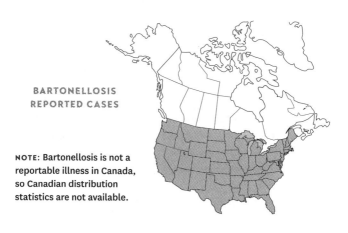

BARTONELLOSIS REPORTED CASES

NOTE: Bartonellosis is not a reportable illness in Canada, so Canadian distribution statistics are not available.

Signs and Symptoms of Bartonellosis

- ✗ Fever
- ✗ Lymph node swelling
- ✗ Headache
- ✗ Bone pain, usually in shins, neck, and back
- ✗ Muscle pain
- ✗ Abdominal pain
- ✗ Pain at the bottom of the feet
- ✗ Rash

The question of whether *Bartonella* species can be transmitted by ticks to humans is a topic demanding serious scientific exploration. In addition, more research is necessary to identify which specific *Bartonella* species is carried by *Ixodes scapularis* and *I. pacificus*. I suspect there will be more research in the near future that will address this important issue.

Tick Paralysis

A RARE PHENOMENON CALLED TICK PARALYSIS can be caused by a neurotoxin carried in the saliva of the deer tick, American dog tick, Rocky Mountain wood tick, and lone star tick. Tick paralysis is the only tick-borne disease that is not caused by a pathogen and that can only persist while the tick is attached. Poor coordination followed by paralysis that starts from the lower parts of the body moving upward, and numbness or tingling, is the common presentation. It usually happens after the tick has been attached for 5 or more days. As soon as the tick is removed, the symptoms resolve.

Emerging Research:
Is Q Fever a Tick-Borne Disease?

Q fever is caused by the bacterium *Coxiella burnetii*, which is most commonly transmitted through the air (by breathing in dust contaminated by the urine, feces, birthing products, or milk of infected goats, sheep, and cattle) but has also been detected in some tick species. Although it has been shown that *C. burnetii* can be transmitted from ticks to vertebrates, it is unknown whether it can cause disease.[24] I suspect there will be more research in the near future to address whether Q fever can be transmitted from ticks to humans and cause disease.

CHAPTER 3

Tick Control and Tick Bite Prevention

Prevention is one of the foundational principles of naturopathic medicine. To end Lyme and tick-borne diseases (TBD), prevention will be key. There are many proactive strategies you may take to prevent Lyme and TBD. We will cover two main categories now: tick population reduction and personal tick bite prevention. This chapter discusses managing and repelling ticks. Subsequent chapters will discuss how to prevent tick-borne disease with prophylactic measures (chapter 4), what to do if you receive a tick bite (chapter 5), and treatments for acute TBD (chapter 6).

Reducing the Tick Population

THE FIRST STRATEGY TO PREVENT LYME and TBD is reducing the tick population. To do so, we must focus on tick hosts as well as ticks themselves. Fortunately, many excellent resources and products address keeping ticks away from your land, out of your home, and away from your body. With tick habitat in mind, altering the landscape, targeting the mouse population, considering outdoor treatment with acaricides (substances toxic to mites or ticks), controlling the deer population, and pet management are the approaches to tick control we will cover in this section.

Landscaping

Becoming aware of tick habitat is the first step. Tick habitat includes grass, low-lying shrubs, and leaf litter. Ticks thrive in high-humidity environments, between grassy and forested areas, in wood piles, in stone walls, and around the perimeter of buildings surrounded by grass. Ticks live where yards border wooded areas, gardens, woodpiles, stone walls, and sheds. They have an affinity for moist areas and the shade. As Richard S. Ostfeld, author of *Lyme Disease: The Ecology of a Complex System*, explains: "Ticks are more abundant in fragmented patches of moist deciduous forests with shrub understories and are less abundant in large continuous forests and coniferous forests."[25]

Take the following steps to make your land less tick-friendly:

- × Rake leaves.
- × Clear brush and debris from grass and gardens.
- × Keep grass short.
- × Trim shrubs and low branches.

×   Create wide, grass-free paths made of wood chips or stone.

×   Remove bird feeders or place them on the perimeter of the land.

Another good strategy is to demarcate border areas, where ticks seem to thrive. You might consider adding a 3-foot-wide strip of stone or wood chips in places where your lawn meets high plant growth or any kind of structure (prime mouse habitat):

×   Between grass and a building structure

×   Between grass and wooded areas

×   Between grass and gardens

×   Around stone walls

×   Remove any trash, litter, or discarded household items from the yard, and contain garbage in sealed bins.

Guinea hens have been known to eat ticks and are often employed with this goal in mind. However, the best animal for the task is the opossum. Richard Ostfeld undertook a study in which he and his colleagues compared the survival rate of deer tick larvae on six different host species: white-footed mice, chipmunks, gray squirrels, opossums, and two kinds of birds. They found that on the mice, 50 percent of the larvae survived to an engorged state and then dropped off their hosts. In comparison, only 3.5 percent of the larvae survived on the opossums; their hosts ate most of the rest. Numbers for the other species fell somewhere in between.[26]

Bird migration is a major cause of the spread of ticks and therefore tick-borne disease throughout the United States and Canada. Removing or moving bird feeders to the perimeter is an appropriate preventive measure to decrease the tick population in your yard.

Reducing Tick Habitat Around Your Home

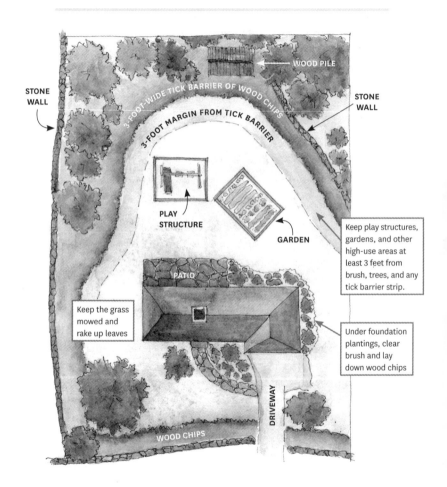

WOOD PILE

STONE WALL

STONE WALL

3-FOOT-WIDE TICK BARRIER OF WOOD CHIPS

3-FOOT MARGIN FROM TICK BARRIER

PLAY STRUCTURE

GARDEN

Keep play structures, gardens, and other high-use areas at least 3 feet from brush, trees, and any tick barrier strip.

PATIO

Keep the grass mowed and rake up leaves

Under foundation plantings, clear brush and lay down wood chips

DRIVEWAY

WOOD CHIPS

Eliminating Barberry

Certain landscaping plants, such as Japanese barberry, may be inadvertently creating prime tick habitat. Japanese barberry (*Berberis thunbergii*) is a small shrub with thin, spiny branches and dense foliage. Native to Asia, it was introduced to the United States as an ornamental plant in the late 1800s and is now considered an invasive species. Japanese barberry is very adaptable and thrives in shaded woodlands, open fields, wetlands — almost anywhere. The seeds are easily spread by birds that eat the red berries from the shrub. Deer do not like Japanese barberry but will eat the other native plants nearby, which allows for the selective proliferation of Japanese barberry.

The map of Japanese barberry distribution in the United States looks a lot like the map of Lyme disease incidence. In fact, deer tick rates are significantly higher in areas with Japanese barberry infestations.[27] Its foliage harbors the perfect humid conditions for ticks to thrive. Mice also enjoy that humidity and build their nests beneath Japanese barberry, where they may provide a tick with its first blood meal infused with *Borrelia burgdorferi*. It has been found that white-footed mice in areas with Japanese barberry have more ticks attached to them, whereas white-footed mice in areas with

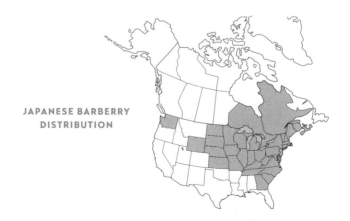

**JAPANESE BARBERRY
DISTRIBUTION**

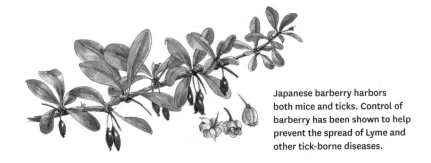

Japanese barberry harbors both mice and ticks. Control of barberry has been shown to help prevent the spread of Lyme and other tick-borne diseases.

less Japanese barberry have fewer attached ticks.[28] For this reason, management of Japanese barberry as a way to prevent the spread of Lyme and other tick-borne disease is imperative.

In fact, the identification, removal, and management of Japanese barberry has been shown to decrease tick populations. Preventing seed production and dispersal is the main goal. Here are some main ways to remove small or shaded areas of Japanese barberry where their shallow roots will lend to easy management:

- ✕ **PULL SEEDLINGS AND SMALL PLANTS.** They are easier to pull when the soil is moist. Use gloves to protect your hands from the spiny branches. Pull slowly and steadily. Remove the root crown in order to prevent resprouting. Pack down soil.

- ✕ **DIG LARGER PLANTS.** Use a spade to remove. Pack down the soil and cover with leaves.

- ✕ **CUT OR MOW.** Done repeatedly, this will limit the spread but not eliminate the plant, as it will resprout.

- ✕ **WRAP THE STUMP.** After cutting, wrap the stumps in burlap or plastic and tie with a rope.

- ✕ **DISPOSE OF PLANTS.** Dry out the plants. Burn or bag the berries.

- ✕ **MONITOR.** Check the areas of removal periodically to control new growth.

Acaricides: Research Continues

Research into acaricides — preparations that kill ticks (and mites) — has not, to date, come up with an effective and safe-for-other-species method of tick control in the landscape. Here's where things stand at the time of this book's publication:

PYRETHROIDS. The most effective way to kill and repel ticks on land is to use pyrethroids. Permethrin and bifenthrin are types of pyrethroids, a host-targeted acaricide. Pyrethroids are synthetic versions of pyrethrins, which come from pyrethrum, the oleoresin extract of dried chrysanthemum flowers. They interfere with the nervous system of insects and arachnids on contact. Pyrethroids are toxic to bumblebees, butterflies, and aquatic life, and moderately toxic to birds. Therefore, I do not feel comfortable recommending pyrethroid use on the landscape.

FUNGAL SPRAYS. A current study called the Tick Project, created by Richard Ostfeld and Felicia Keesing, is under way evaluating efficacy of a product called the Tick Control System and a natural alternative, the Met52 fungal spray (both are commercially available).[29] The Tick Control System is a box with bait that attracts small mammals and dispenses a dose of fipronil, a pyrethroid, onto the animal. The fungus being studied is *Metarhizium anisopliae* strain F52, which offers a natural alternative to pyrethroids. Studies have shown that the fungal spray Met52 causes a decrease of nymphal deer ticks by 55 percent on lawns and 85 percent on woodland plots.[30] Fungus spores attach and penetrate the outer surface of the tick, then grow inside the tick, causing the tick to die. It does not harm birds, mammals, bees, or aquatic wildlife and is nontoxic to humans.

ESSENTIAL OILS. In addition to fungal spray, there are other natural alternatives to using pyrethroids. Desiccants like diatomaceous earth have not been shown to be effective. Essential oils, though, have shown some promise. Certain essential oils have been shown to repel or be toxic to ticks.[31] Cedar, rosemary, peppermint, and wintergreen essential oils are among those showing good results. Studies of a commercially available essential oil formulation suggest that a high-pressure spray is more effective than a low-pressure one (probably because it has a better saturation rate).

Nootkatone, a sesquiterpene found in the essential oil of grapefruit and the heartwood of yellow cedar (*Xanthocyparis nootkatensis* or *Chamaecyparis nootkatensis*), has been shown to be most effective as a tick repellent. Researchers are currently testing different nootkatone formulations in an effort to identify those that will last long enough to serve as a tick-control spray outside. The challenge of achieving long-lasting efficacy (and the variations in efficacy shown in the literature) may be related to the specific formulation of the essential oils with other ingredients, environmental conditions, and application method.

. . .

At the time of this writing, I do not have a specific recommendation for a safe and effective acaricide treatment for the land. Unfortunately, traditional pyrethroids continue to be the most effective available intervention. As more research is completed, however, I expect a safe and effective natural alternative to be available in the near future.

Targeting Mice: Tick Tubes

The next step in tick control is addressing the animals that act as hosts to ticks. As Richard Ostfeld explains, "White footed mice are consistently shown to be the most efficient wildlife reservoirs of *Borrelia burgdorferi*, infecting between 75 and 95 percent of larval blacklegged ticks that feed on them."[32] Wood piles, brush piles, compost piles, stone walls, and rotting wood will attract mice. Eliminating or limiting these areas is a key step.

Tick tubes are an excellent intervention to target ticks in areas where mice nest. Place these biodegradable cardboard tubes filled with permethrin-treated cotton in areas where mice are found. The mice will take the permethrin-treated cotton to build their nests. The permethrin will not harm the mice or other animals, but it will kill ticks and, most important, at the larval stage. It is the larvae that most often feed on mice, and the permethrin kills them before they have a chance to acquire pathogens from the mice and before they reach the nymph and adult stages, when they might use humans as hosts. Research shows that over an 8-year period, there was on average a 93.6 percent reduction in exposure per hour to infected ticks in treated areas of the Fire Island Pines, New York.[33] I hear reports of successful tick reduction from patients of mine who have treated their land with tick tubes. After applying tick tubes, many people have shared that they went from finding many ticks one year to finding few or no ticks on their property the next year.

You can purchase tick tubes from farm stores and online (see Resources). You can also make your own tick tubes; see below.

Set out the tick tubes in early spring, midsummer, and early fall to target the surges in tick numbers as a result of the tick life cycle. Use six tick tubes per ⅛ acre of mouse habitat. To calculate mouse habitat, do not include buildings, paved areas, or lawn. Place the tubes in mouse habitat: wood piles, stone walls, near compost, around the perimeter of structures like a shed, under bushes, and in gardens. If possible, place the tubes in places that would stay dry when it rains. Space the tubes 30 feet away from each other. You may replace the tubes when you notice they are empty. If you notice that tubes are remaining full, consider moving them a few inches or feet in one direction or another to improve the potential for mice to find them.

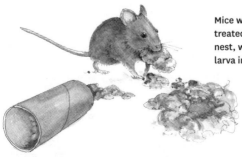

Mice will take the permethrin-treated cotton back to their nest, where it will kill any tick larva infesting the nest.

Make Your Own Tick Tubes

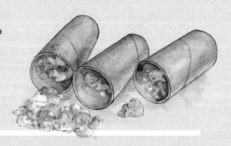

YOU WILL NEED

- Permethrin (available at sporting good stores, farm stores, and so on); it comes in spray form or as a concentrated liquid

- Spray bottle (if your permethrin solution is not already in a spray bottle)

- Cotton balls, old cotton batting from cushions or pillows, even old dryer lint — any fluffy natural material that will degrade over time

- Gloves and a mask

- Cardboard box

- Cardboard tubes from toilet paper or paper towel rolls

NOTE: Keep the permethrin away from your skin and pets while wet. It is safe to touch once dried. And remember that permethrin is toxic to bumblebees, butterflies, and aquatic life; be sure that when you are spraying the permethrin, the spray will not drift onto any nearby plants or into waterways. The permethrin does not cause an environmental concern because it binds tightly with the fiber in the tubes. If for some reason permethrin did come into contact with soil, it degrades quickly, so it will not seep into groundwater.

1 If you're working with concentrated permethrin, dilute it, following the instructions on the packaging, and pour it into a spray bottle.

2 Put on your gloves and mask.

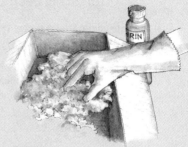

STEP 3

3 Lay out the cotton or lint in the box. Set the box in a well-ventilated area.

4 Spray the cotton or lint with the permethrin, soaking it thoroughly. Flip it over and spray the other side.

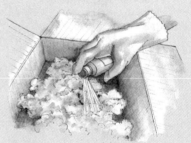

STEP 4

5 Let the cotton or lint dry for a few hours.

6 Stuff the permethrin-treated cotton or lint into the cardboard tubes, leaving the last inch or so of the ends empty.

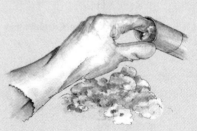

STEP 6

Targeting Deer: Deer-Resistant Plants

Deer are common tick hosts. They enjoy grassy or leafy areas and will feed on Japanese yews, honeysuckle, and fruit trees. To reduce deer traffic in your yard, use high, sturdy fencing and add plants to your garden that deer will tend to find unpalatable.

Northeast

Bee balm	Lungwort
Brunnera	Meadow rue
Catmint	Sea holly
Golden marguerite	Sweet woodruff
Jack in the pulpit	Turtlehead
Japanese painted fern	Virginia bluebells
Lily of the valley	Wild ginger

Midwest

Amsonia	Globe thistle
Bugbane	Lungwort
Butterfly weed	Penstemon
Columbine	Purple coneflower
Coreopsis	Russian sage
Corydalis	Thyme
Evening primrose	Wild ginger

Mountain West and High Plains

Ajuga	Penstemon
Allium	Purple coneflower
Candytuft	Russian sage
Coralbells	Salvia
Coreopsis	Shasta daisy
Globe thistle	Wormwood
Hens and chicks	Yucca
Ornamental grasses	

South

Bear's breeches	Goldenrod
Butterfly weed	Hens and chicks
Caryopteris	Joe-pye weed
Chrysanthemum	New Zealand flax
Crocosmia	Red-hot poker
Dianthus	Rosemary
Epimedium	Russian sage

Pacific Northwest

Bellflower	Lupine
Bigroot geranium	Meadow rue
Corydalis	Mullein
Epimedium	Oregano
Foxglove	Pigsqueak
Jerusalem sage	Yellow wax bells
Ligularia	

Southwest

Agave	Rosemary
Blanketflower	Soapwort
California fuchsia	Snow-in-summer
Hedgehog cactus	Society garlic
Lavender	Texas sage
Lavender cotton	Yucca
Oriental poppy	

Southern California

Agave	Rosemary
Blanketflower	Shasta daisy
California fuchsia	Soapwort
Hedgehog cactus	Snow-in-summer
Hens and chicks	Society garlic
Lavender	Texas sage
Lavender cotton	Yucca
Oriental poppy	

Pet Management

Owning a pet that goes outdoors increases your tick bite risk because your pet can carry the tick back to you or your home. One study showed that pet owners had almost twice the risk of finding ticks crawling on them and about one and a half times the risk of finding ticks attached to them.[34] Consider using fencing to keep wildlife out and your dog from going into tick habitat. Groom pets and conduct tick checks after possible tick exposure. Use a lint roller on their fur to help. Recognize the areas of the home where outdoor pets occupy. Consider limiting your outdoor pets' presence in sleeping and living areas of the house.

The following pet products kill ticks before they bite: Seresto collar (flumethrin and imidacloprid; safe for cats and dogs), K9 Advantix II (permethrin and imidacloprid; safe for dogs only), and Vectra 3D (dinotefuran, pyriproxyfen, and permethrin; safe for dogs only). You may also have your dog wear a bandana or shirt treated with permethrin; you can buy one from Insect Shield (see Resources) or treat the bandana or shirt yourself (see page 80). There are lots of other products, most of which are safe for dogs and some that are safe for cats, that will kill ticks but not necessarily before they bite your pet. Many other options are discussed by the TickEncounter Resource Center.[35] Your best bet for tick-control pet products is your local veterinarian.

As an alternative to the above chemical products, you may also use the tick-repellent spray made of cedarwood oil called Cedarcide Tickshield on dogs. I also highly recommend treating any materials that your pets regularly lie on, like a dog bed, with permethrin to kill ticks that come indoors with pets. The next section will outline these options in detail.

Personal Tick Bite Prevention Strategies

THE SECOND STRATEGY FOR PREVENTING LYME and TBD is using personal tick bite prevention strategies. It is important to know how to keep ticks off yourself, especially when you are in locations where tick-management strategies may not be in place.

Here are effective strategies for those times when you're in tick territory:

× Use personal tick repellent (see page 79).

× Wear permethrin-treated clothing (see page 80).

× Wear light-colored clothing.

× Tuck pants into socks and shirts into pants.

× Avoid walking through grass and leaf litter.

× Treat your pets with tick-control products, and check them for ticks every few hours while outdoors and when they come indoors.

× When you come in from the outdoors, place your clothes directly in the dryer on high heat for 6 minutes to kill ticks. (If you choose to wash your clothes first, the water temperature must be equal to or greater than 130°F/54°C) in order to kill nymph and adult deer ticks. If the water temperature is below 130°F/54°C, only 50 percent of the ticks will be killed by washing, and the rest will have benefited from being saturated. You'll have to dry those clothes in a dryer on high heat for 55 minutes to kill the remaining ticks.)[36]

× Shower soon after coming indoors. (Note: This in and of itself will not wash off attached ticks, but it will aid you in spotting them and may wash off crawling ticks.)

× Conduct a full-body tick check (see page 78).

Tick Check!

Use sight and touch to sense for any ticks crawling on or attached to your entire body. Ticks are attracted to warmth and moisture, so make sure to search under your arms, behind your knees, between your legs, inside your belly button, between your buttocks, in your genitals, under your bra, around your waist, around and in your ears, on your head, and between your toes. Use a mirror or another set of eyes to check hard-to-see places.

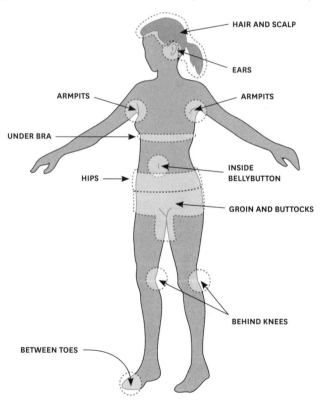

HAIR AND SCALP

EARS

ARMPITS

ARMPITS

UNDER BRA

INSIDE BELLYBUTTON

HIPS

GROIN AND BUTTOCKS

BEHIND KNEES

BETWEEN TOES

Deer Tick Season

Deer ticks are generally thought of as a summertime pest, but these ticks — the primary vector for Lyme disease — are active anytime temperatures are above 28°F (–2°C). Take steps to protect yourself whenever temperatures are above this baseline.

Personal Tick Repellent

While research is not conclusive about the effectiveness of using essential oils on the land, research and experience shows that essential oils on the skin are effective as a personal tick-repellent spray while we are in tick habitat. The product I recommend and use myself is called Cedarcide Tickshield, which is 20 percent cedarwood oil and 80 percent hydrated silica. Cedarwood oil disrupts the ticks' pheromones, which interferes with bodily functions like breathing and disorients the tick. In one study, when deer ticks were placed on the bottom of filter paper that was treated with Tickshield on the top half and held in a vertical direction, 100 percent of the ticks were repelled.[37] Tickshield is also safe as a repellent on dogs over 20 pounds, but it is not safe for cats. I recommend Tickshield for human use as the primary repellent. It is safe to spray generously on your skin, clothing, and head to repel ticks. I recommend reapplying every 1 to 2 hours. It is nontoxic to bees, butterflies, and fish.

As we learned in our discussion of acaricides (page 69), nootkatone — a constituent in the essential oil of grapefruit and the heartwood of yellow cedar — has been shown to repel deer ticks[38] and is safe to use on human skin. One study showed that nootkatone provided 100 percent repellence of adult deer ticks and lone star ticks for 3 days.[39] Although the CDC has entered into a licensing agreement with Evolva to develop a commercially available tick repellent for public use, nootkatone is not yet commercially available.

Tick-Repellent Clothing

As mentioned earlier, permethrin is a pyrethroid acaricide. While I do not recommend spraying permethrin on the land, I do recommend its careful use in treating materials. Permethrin-treated clothing and gear is highly effective against tick bites and safe for use. In one study, researchers reported that "subjects wearing permethrin-treated sneakers and socks were 73.6 times less likely to have a tick bite than subjects wearing untreated footwear."[40]

If you would like to treat your clothes and gear with permethrin, you may do it yourself or send your clothes away to a company that applies permethrin commercially.

AT-HOME TREATMENT

For do-it-yourself projects, there are two common brands available: Sawyer (0.5 percent permethrin) and Martin's (10 percent permethrin). It is recommended to treat materials like clothing, shoes, and gear using 0.5 percent permethrin. The treatment will be effective through 6 washes, or 6 weeks. Martin's 10 percent permethrin is a concentrated option that must be diluted before use. Use 1 part Martin's 10 percent permethrin to 19 parts water to create a 0.5 percent permethrin solution.

When treating clothes with permethrin yourself, make sure to do so outside, away from children and pets, while wearing gloves to protect your skin. Remember that in liquid form, permethrin is toxic to human skin and pets. It is safe when it has dried. There are two methods of application: the spray method and the soak method. If you are treating shoes, socks, hats, gloves, or a small amount of material, I recommend using the spray method. Spray 0.5 percent permethrin directly onto clothing and gear with a slow, sweeping motion, keeping the bottle 6 to 8 inches away from the cloth. Treat each side of the piece of clothing for 30 seconds, or until the item is saturated.[41] After applying permethrin, hang clothing or gear to dry for 2 to 4 hours. I especially recommend using this method to treat shoes, boots, and sneakers every 6 weeks.

For a larger amount of clothing or for bulky clothing, I recommend sending the items to a commercial permethrin applicator, but you can also use the soak method to do it yourself. Lightly roll up the clothing being treated and place it in a 1-gallon resealable bag. Pour enough 0.5 percent permethrin into the bag to cover the clothing. Sawyer recommends using 3 ounces of formula per garment. Seal the bag and move the solution around inside bag to ensure the clothing is soaked. Remove excess air and reseal the bag. Let the bag stand for 2 hours. Remove treated clothing and hang to dry.

COMMERICAL TREATMENT

Of course, you can buy clothes that have already been treated with permethrin, but if you have clothing that you *wish* were treated, there are companies that will do it for you. I recommend Insect Shield (see Resources), which has created a factory-based technique for long-lasting permethrin impregnation of clothing that allows for clothes to hold their pesticidal activity against *Ixodes scapularis* (deer ticks) for 70 washes.[42] A study conducted on workers from the North Carolina Division of Water Quality wearing clothing treated by Insect Shield found a 99 percent decrease in the rate of tick bites acquired during work hours and a 93 percent decrease in the total incidence of tick bites.[43] It has also been shown that Insect Shield technology does not emit any odor that alarms deer, which will be of particular interest to hunters.[44]

Ultimately, your best approach is to utilize both methods of commercial permethrin application and home treatment to create a comprehensive safeguard against ticks. Send clothing, blankets, sheets, and gear for commercial application of permethrin, and treat shoes every 6 weeks with permethrin at home. Be aware that dry cleaning removes permethrin from clothing. And store permethrin-treated clothing in darkness to reduce deterioration from UV light.

CHAPTER 4

Herbal Prophylaxis for Lyme and Tick-Borne Disease

Implementing tick bite prevention strategies is crucial, but equally important is knowing when to administer prophylaxis — that is, a measure taken to prevent disease. Prophylactic measures can be initiated by anyone immediately after finding a tick bite, and they can be used regularly by people at high risk for tick bites. This chapter explores the importance of prophylaxis, identifies which herbal formulas can be used as prophylaxis for which types of tick bites, and examines the herbs used to make the formulas.

Why Prophylaxis?

I BELIEVE THAT PROPHYLAXIS IS IMPORTANT because it can be so difficult to diagnose Lyme and other tick-borne disease (TBD) properly. Prophylaxis allows you to take measures to treat illness preemptively, before it even manifests as symptoms in your body. The philosophy is not unique to tick-borne diseases. For example, people who are going to visit regions where malaria is endemic are encouraged to take a prophylactic pharmaceutical regimen, before they travel, to protect themselves just in case they are bitten by a mosquito that transmits the protozoan that causes malaria. Better to treat ahead of time rather than wait for symptoms and diagnosis.

The same holds true for Lyme and other TBD. Whether you are bitten by a tick or simply living, working, or recreating in an area where these diseases are endemic, you can take measures to prevent infection with these diseases. My preference for the prophylactic approach is based on several factors regarding Lyme and TBD diagnostics:

× Fewer than 50 percent of people with Lyme disease remember receiving a tick bite.

× Fewer than 50 percent of people with Lyme disease see a bull's-eye rash.

× Symptoms of Lyme disease may take 30 days or more to develop after a tick bite.

× Conventional Lyme disease and babesiosis testing is not reliable.

× There are no testing options for TBD like those caused by certain *Borrelia* species and STARI at the time of this writing.

× More *Borrelia* species and other pathogens that cause TBD are being discovered almost every year.

With such ambiguity and a lack of easy and accurate detection, prophylaxis is the best way to protect yourself against the development

Conventional Prophylaxis: Doxycycline

The conventional recommendation for a single dose of doxycycline after a tick bite is based primarily on one study from 2001. From a population of people who had received a tick bite within the preceding 72 hours, researchers created one group who received doxycycline and one group who received a placebo. They concluded that the doxycycline significantly reduced the development of Lyme disease.[45] However, the definition of Lyme disease used in this study was confined to the development of an erythema migrans rash. The researchers did not evaluate other manifestations of Lyme disease, such as fever, viral-like illness, or erythema migrans at sites other than the tick bite, though those symptoms were documented in some members of the doxycycline group. Therefore, in my opinion this study does not provide evidence that a single dose of doxycycline will prevent you from developing Lyme disease manifesting without an erythema migrans. Most importantly, I have seen many patients exhibit symptoms of Lyme disease even after taking a single 200 mg dose of doxycycline prescribed by another health care provider for a tick bite.

of TBD. Starting herbal antibiotic prophylaxis immediately after a tick bite (or having it already in your system — see the following discussion of prophylaxis for high-risk populations) activates the immune system and initiates an antimicrobial response that will help destroy any pathogens that may be transmitted to you from the tick.

I prefer herbal antimicrobials over pharmaceutical antibiotic prophylaxis for a number of reasons. First, antibiotics only kill bacteria. Some TBDs, being protozoa or viruses, require different treatments. The herbal prophylactic formulas are designed to address all possible pathogens carried by a specific tick. Unlike pharmaceutical antibiotics, which often contain just one chemical compound that is engineered to kill certain classes of bacteria in a certain way, plants are complex and have many chemical compounds that synergize in favor of our bodies and against the pathogens. Herbs help our immune system function better in the face of tick-borne pathogens, do not negatively impact gut flora, have fewer side effects, and are safe to take long-term. At this stage of treatment, when there is no known infection, I recommend avoiding pharmaceutical use and opting for a prophylactic herbal approach. (It's safe to take both a pharmaceutical antibiotic and an herbal antimicrobial formula at the same time.)

The prophylactic herbal antimicrobial formulas in this book are designed to target specific pathogens. While the most common tick-borne disease in the United States is Lyme disease, caused by *Borrelia burgdorferi*, other tick-borne pathogens must be prevented, too. As we reviewed earlier, there are many different types of ticks, and each can carry various pathogens. By looking at the geographic area in which you reside, work, or visit, you may determine which ticks are endemic and, therefore, for which pathogens you are at risk.

Prophylaxis for High-Risk Populations

EVERY STATE AND PROVINCE in the United States and Canada has at least one tick species native to its landscape that causes human disease (see the chart on pages 170–171). So everyone is at risk for a tick bite, but some people are at higher risk than others. Some occupations and hobbies lend themselves to higher tick exposure. Spending more time in tick habitat increases the likelihood of a tick bite, and therefore tick-borne disease.

Occupations and pastimes in which you are consistently exposed to prime tick habitat or in contact with animals that are consistently exposed to prime tick habitat increase your risk for a tick bite. They include:

- ✗ Farming
- ✗ Landscaping
- ✗ Electrical line work
- ✗ Work with animals (including veterinary medicine)
- ✗ Logging
- ✗ Land surveying
- ✗ Construction
- ✗ Forestry
- ✗ Railroad work
- ✗ Oil field work
- ✗ Park and wildlife management
- ✗ Hiking, camping, or fishing
- ✗ Gardening or yard work
- ✗ Golfing or playing field sports
- ✗ Stacking or carrying firewood
- ✗ Horseback riding

If you fall into any of these categories, you may want to take additional precautions during tick season. This may include taking an herbal tick bite formula prophylactically — and not only as a response to a tick bite to ward off the potential transmission of TBD, but as part of your daily routine, under the assumption that you *will* be bitten by a tick at some point, and as noted above, many people who are diagnosed with TBD do not remember ever receiving a tick bite.

Taking an herbal antimicrobial formula daily prepares your immune system for defense against your likely exposure to TBD. For example, if you live in an area where Lyme disease is prevalent and you spend a great deal of time in prime tick habitat, you might take the prophylactic tick-bite formula designed for deer ticks (page 91) during high tick season. If you are then bitten by a deer tick infected with *Borrelia burgdorferi*, whether you are aware of the tick bite or not, the herbs have already activated your immune system and a targeted antibacterial mechanism is already at work in your body in order to decrease your chance of becoming infected. This approach allows for the earliest intervention.

As you'll see in the formulas later in this chapter, the dosage for the use of the prophylactic herbal formulas as TBD prevention for high-risk populations is less than the dosage you would take after a known tick bite. The lesser dosage arises from the expectation that the formula will have more of an impact on the incoming pathogens from a tick bite because it will already be in your system. It is safe to take these herbal formulas long-term.

It's important to take the formula that is appropriate for your geographical location. To determine which one(s) are appropriate for you, refer to chapter 1. Consult the maps that display the location of each tick species to determine which ticks pose you the most risk. Confirm that information for your specific location by checking in with your local department of health or cooperative extension office to find out which ticks are transmitting diseases locally. Then look up the formula specific to those particular ticks in the section following.

For example, a farmer in Vermont would consult the maps of tick location and find that deer, brown dog, American dog, and lone star ticks can be found in that state. When the farmer reaches out to the local department of health or agricultural extension office, she or he would find that 99 percent of tick-borne disease in Vermont is transmitted by the deer tick. Historically, the brown dog tick has not transmitted any pathogens in Vermont. At the time of this writing, American dog ticks do not carry disease in Vermont, and although the lone star tick has been reported in Vermont, it is not considered to be established there. So, if the farmer, whose occupation carries a high risk for tick exposure, wishes to protect her- or himself against tick-borne disease, the tick to focus on would be the deer tick, as the primary vector of Lyme disease, and the farmer could take the formula designed for deer tick bites (page 91).

The Prophylactic Tick Bite Formulas

THE PROPHYLACTIC TICK BITE FORMULAS that I use in my practice arose from a collaboration with longtime herbalist Bonnie Bloom of Blue Crow Botanicals in western Massachusetts. Drawing from my clinical experience, Bonnie's herbal expertise, and the research of master herbalist Stephen Harrod Buhner, I first designed an herbal formula to target the pathogens commonly carried by deer ticks, which are widespread in the Northeast, where I practice. After observing the effectiveness of this formula with my patients, I went on to design a series of prophylactic formulas targeting a range of pathogens carried by ticks across the United States and Canada today.

The key herbs used in the prophylactic formulas are discussed in more depth beginning on page 107. They each have specific antimicrobial actions. Their combined effects create immune modulation.

These prophylactic tick bite formulas are multi-herb tinctures — that is, alcohol-based extracts of specific herbs used in combination. In the Resources section (page 180), you'll find details on some trustworthy suppliers from whom you can buy good-quality tinctures. A couple of them offer these exact multi-herb formulas; others offer single-herb tinctures that you can combine in the ratios given in the formulas. If you want to make your own tinctures (see page 102), the Resources section also offers details on which companies are the best sources for herbs.

The dosage of these formulas depends on what you are using them for. If you are at high risk for a tick bite and want antimicrobial protection during tick season (for deer ticks, whenever outdoor temperatures are above 28°F/−2°C), you will need only about half the usual dosage to discourage tick-borne pathogens from establishing an infection.

If you receive a tick bite, prophylactic treatment calls for the full dosage. In addition, I recommend using a natural biofilm buster like serrapeptase at 120,000 units (or 500 mg) twice daily on an empty stomach; see the herbal prophylactic protocol in chapter 5 for more details.

The formulas should be taken on an empty stomach, which means 30 minutes before food and 2 hours after food. If you are unable to use alcohol-based herbal extracts, Woodland Essence (see Resources) has each of the single herbs used in the tick bite formulas available as a glycerite (a glycerin-based herbal extract), except for andrographis. Consult a trained holistic health-care professional if you plan to take a tick bite formula for more than 3 months for further guidance on dosing, side effects, drug interactions, contraindications, and pertinent medical history.

Index of Key Herbs

I refer to the plants used in the prophylactic formulas by their Latin name, rather than their common name, because it is a more specific identifier. Plants can have multiple common names, and a common name can be used for more than one plant. *Houttuynia cordata*, for example, can be called houttuynia, chameleon plant, or bishop's weed, among other common names. And the common name *sage* can be used to refer to many of the plants in the *Salvia* genus, including the species *Salvia miltiorrhiza*, which I use in some of the prophylactic formulas.

In contrast, the Latin name designates just a single species.

LATIN NAME	COMMON NAME
Andrographis paniculata	Andrographis
Cordyceps militaris	Cordyceps, orange caterpillar fungus
Cordyceps sinensis	Cordyceps
Cryptolepis sanguinolenta	Cryptolepis
Houttuynia cordata	Houttuynia, chamelon plant, bishop's weed
Polygonum cuspidatum	Japanese knotweed
Salvia miltiorrhiza	Red sage, dan shen
Scutellaria baicalensis	Chinese skullcap

Deer Tick Bite Formula

- 1 part *Cryptolepis sanguinolenta* root tincture
- 1 part *Houttuynia cordata* fresh aerial parts tincture
- 1 part *Polygonum cuspidatum* root tincture
- 1 part *Uncaria tomentosa* inner vine bark tincture

PREVENTIVE DOSAGE FOR HIGH-RISK POPULATIONS: Take ½ teaspoon of tincture in water three times a day, 30 minutes before breakfast, lunch, and dinner, during tick season.

DOSAGE AFTER A KNOWN TICK BITE: Take 1 teaspoon of tincture in water three times a day, 30 minutes before breakfast, lunch, and dinner, for 30 days. Also take 120,000 units (or 500 mg) of serrapeptase twice daily on an empty stomach.

TARGET PATHOGENS: *Borrelia burgdorferi*, *B. mayonii*, *B. miyamotoi*, *Babesia* species, *Anaplasma phagocytophilum*, *Ehrlichia muris eauclairensis*, and Powassan virus

NOTE: I use a different prophylactic protocol for deer tick bites in children; see page 98.

American Dog Tick Bite Formula

- 3 parts *Polygonum cuspidatum* root tincture
- 1 part *Cryptolepis sanguinolenta* root tincture
- 1 part *Salvia miltiorrhiza* root tincture
- 1 part *Scutellaria baicalensis* root tincture

PREVENTIVE DOSAGE FOR HIGH-RISK POPULATIONS: Take ½ teaspoon of tincture in water three times a day, 30 minutes before breakfast, lunch, and dinner, during tick season.

DOSAGE AFTER A KNOWN TICK BITE: Take 1 teaspoon of tincture in water three times a day, 30 minutes before breakfast, lunch, and dinner, for 30 days. Also take 120,000 units (or 500 mg) of serrapeptase twice daily on an empty stomach.

TARGET PATHOGENS: *Rickettsia rickettsii* and *Francisella tularensis*

Lone Star Tick Bite Formula

- 1 part *Cryptolepis sanguinolenta* root tincture
- 1 part *Houttuynia cordata* aerial parts tincture
- 1 part *Polygonum cuspidatum* root tincture
- 1 part *Salvia miltiorrhiza* root tincture
- 1 part *Uncaria tomentosa* bark tincture

PREVENTIVE DOSAGE FOR HIGH-RISK POPULATIONS: Take 5/8 teaspoon of tincture in water three times a day, 30 minutes before breakfast, lunch, and dinner, during tick season.

DOSAGE AFTER A KNOWN TICK BITE: Take 1¼ teaspoons of tincture in water three times a day, 30 minutes before breakfast, lunch, and dinner, for 30 days. Also take 120,000 units (or 500 mg) of serrapeptase twice daily on an empty stomach.

TARGET PATHOGENS/DISEASES: STARI, *Ehrlichia chaffeensis*, *E. ewingii*, Heartland virus, *Francisella tularensis*

Brown Dog Tick Bite Formula

- 3 parts *Polygonum cuspidatum* root tincture
- 1 part *Cordyceps militaris* or *C. sinensis* tincture
- 1 part *Salvia miltiorrhiza* root tincture
- 1 part *Scutellaria baicalensis* root tincture

PREVENTIVE DOSAGE FOR HIGH-RISK POPULATIONS: Take ½ teaspoon of tincture in water three times a day, 30 minutes before breakfast, lunch, and dinner, during tick season.

DOSAGE AFTER A KNOWN TICK BITE: Take 1 teaspoon of tincture in water three times a day, 30 minutes before breakfast, lunch, and dinner, for 30 days. Also take 120,000 units (or 500 mg) of serrapeptase twice daily on an empty stomach.

TARGET PATHOGEN: *Rickettsia rickettsii*

Gulf Coast Tick Bite Formula

- 3 parts *Polygonum cuspidatum* root tincture
- 1 part *Houttuynia cordata* aerial parts tincture
- 1 part *Salvia miltiorrhiza* root tincture
- 1 part *Scutellaria baicalensis* root tincture

....

PREVENTIVE DOSAGE FOR HIGH-RISK POPULATIONS: Take ½ teaspoon of tincture in water three times a day, 30 minutes before breakfast, lunch, and dinner, during tick season.

DOSAGE AFTER A KNOWN TICK BITE: Take 1 teaspoon of tincture in water three times a day, 30 minutes before breakfast, lunch, and dinner, for 30 days. Also take 120,000 units (or 500 mg) of serrapeptase twice daily on an empty stomach.

....

TARGET PATHOGENS: *Rickettsia parkeri* and *Ehrlichia chaffeensis*

Rocky Mountain Wood Tick Bite Formula

- 3 parts *Polygonum cuspidatum* root tincture
- 1 part *Cryptolepis sanguinolenta* root tincture
- 1 part *Houttuynia cordata* aerial parts tincture
- 1 part *Salvia miltiorrhiza* root tincture
- 1 part *Scutellaria baicalensis* root tincture

PREVENTIVE DOSAGE FOR HIGH-RISK POPULATIONS: Take ⅝ teaspoon of tincture in water three times a day, 30 minutes before breakfast, lunch, and dinner, during tick season.

DOSAGE AFTER A KNOWN TICK BITE: Take 1¼ teaspoons of tincture in water three times a day, 30 minutes before breakfast, lunch, and dinner, for 30 days. Also take 120,000 units (or 500 mg) of serrapeptase twice daily on an empty stomach.

TARGET PATHOGENS: *Rickettsia rickettsii, Francisella tularensis,* and Colorado tick fever virus

Ornithodoros Tick Bite Formula

- 1 part *Andrographis paniculata* aerial parts tincture
- 1 part *Polygonum cuspidatum* root tincture
- 1 part *Uncaria rhynchophylla* inner vine bark tincture
- 1 part *Uncaria tomentosa* inner vine bark tincture

PREVENTIVE DOSAGE FOR HIGH-RISK POPULATIONS: Take ½ teaspoon of tincture in water three times a day, 30 minutes before breakfast, lunch, and dinner, during tick season.

DOSAGE AFTER A KNOWN TICK BITE: Take 1 teaspoon of tincture in water three times a day, 30 minutes before breakfast, lunch, and dinner, for 30 days. Also take 120,000 units (or 500 mg) of serrapeptase twice daily on an empty stomach.

TARGET PATHOGENS: *Borrelia hermsii*, *B. parkeri*, and *B. turicatae*

Prophylactic Protocols for Children

AN ALTERNATIVE DEER TICK BITE FORMULA

The herbs in the deer tick bite formula on page 91, especially cryptolepis, are very bitter, and therefore children are sometimes resistant to taking it. I typically use a different prophylactic protocol with children in my practice, which leads to better compliance because it tastes better. All of the products called for in this protocol come from Nutramedix, a nutraceutical company offering both herbs and supplements; see the Resources section.

The protocol for deer tick bites includes the following:

HOUTTUYNIA: Combats *Anaplasma*, *Ehrlichia*, Powassan virus, and *Bartonella* species. The adult dosage is 30 drops in water 30 minutes before breakfast, lunch, and dinner; adjust the dosage based on the child's weight.

MORA: Contains blackberry, capirona, and yarrow, which combat *Babesia* species. The adult dosage is 30 drops in water 30 minutes before breakfast, lunch, and dinner; adjust the dosage based on the child's weight.

SAMENTO: Contains *Uncaria tomentosa* and works against the Lyme spirochete and round body forms. The adult dosage is 30 drops in water 30 minutes before breakfast, lunch, and dinner; adjust the dosage based on the child's weight.

SERRAPEPTASE: A biofilm buster. The Nutramedix capsule contains 500 mg. The dosage depends on your child's weight:

×   Up to 37 pounds: ½ capsule 30 minutes before breakfast

×   38–75 pounds: ½ capsule 30 minutes before breakfast and dinner

- ✕ 76–112 pounds: 1 capsule 30 minutes before breakfast and ½ capsule 30 minutes before dinner

- ✕ 113+ pounds: 1 capsule 30 minutes before breakfast and dinner

If your child does not swallow capsules or if the dose is half a capsule, open the serrapeptase capsule and pour out the powder. It can be taken directly or mixed into applesauce (or a similar food). It does not stir into liquid very well. Do not put it into a food containing protein (like yogurt), as the serrapeptase would then work on breaking down the protein rather than the biofilm.

ADJUSTING DOSAGES FOR CHILDREN

The tincture dosages given in this book are for an average adult of approximately 150 pounds. In order to calculate the correct dosage for a child, we will use Clark's rule:

$$\frac{\text{Child's weight}}{150 \text{ pounds}} = \frac{\text{Child's dose}}{\text{Stated adult dose}}$$

For example, if a child weighs 50 pounds and the stated adult dose of a preparation is 30 drops:

$$\frac{50 \text{ pounds}}{150 \text{ pounds}} = \frac{x \text{ drops}}{30 \text{ drops}}$$

$$50 \div 150 = 0.3333$$

$$0.3333 = x \div 30$$

$$0.3333 \times 30 = x$$

$$10 \text{ drops} = x$$

The child's dose is 10 drops.

Make Your Own Tick Bite Prophylactic Tincture

In this section, we will focus on the tincture used to treat deer tick bites, which is the prophylactic formula we use most commonly in my practice. You could use these instructions as a template for making the other tick bite formulas as well.

A tincture is an alcohol extract of dried or fresh plants with medicinal properties. The alcohol is part of the menstruum, the liquid solvent that pulls active constituents from the plants soaking in it. The alcohol makes up a specific percentage of the menstruum, while the rest is made up of water and sometimes a small amount of apple cider vinegar. To prepare a tincture, you must know the ratio of the total weight of herbs to the volume of the menstruum. For the deer tick bite formula, we will use a ratio of 1:5 for dried plants and 1:2 or 1:3 for fresh plants:

× In a 1:5 tincture, 100 grams of herb is used per 500 mL of menstruum.

× In a 1:2 tincture, 150 grams of herb is used per 300 mL of menstruum.

× In a 1:3 herb tincture, 100 grams of herb is used per 300 mL of menstruum.

I have deep appreciation and respect for Bonnie Bloom's work as an herbalist. She has humbly given me permission to share her instructions on how to make deer tick bite formula. Making this formula is not simple! To obtain the level of medicinal value I expect in a formula like this, I recommend that you either follow these directions exactly or purchase the tinctures from a trusted source (see page 180).

SUPPLIES

- Mortar and pestle, very clean coffee grinder, blender, or Vitamix high-speed blender
- *Cryptolepis sanguinolenta*: 100 grams of dried root
- *Houttuynia cordata*: 150 grams of fresh aerial parts (or 100 grams of dried aerial parts)
- *Polygonum cuspidatum*: 100 grams of dried root (or if freshly dug, 100 grams of fresh root)
- *Uncaria tomentosa*: 100 grams of dry bark
- Scale
- Measuring cup or measuring cylinder
- 8 widemouthed quart jars with tight-fitting lids
- 190-proof ethyl alcohol
- Spring water
- Apple cider vinegar
- Spoon
- Cotton T-shirt or polyester material
- Rubber gloves

Acidity of Water

In making your own tincture, it is helpful to know the pH of your water. The most important active constituents in cat's claw and cryptolepis are water-soluble alkaloids, which require an acidic pH to dissolve in water. One option is to test your water with a pH test strip. On a scale of 1 (acid) to 14 (alkaline), the pH needs to be 6 or less to allow for the extraction of the alkaloids. If the water used during the extraction process is alkaline, the constituents will not dissolve well. Adding apple cider vinegar to alkaline water will make it more acidic. If you do not know the pH of your water or if you know it is alkaline, use apple cider vinegar to ensure acidity.

Because those alkaloids are so important to the action of cat's claw and cryptolepis, the menstruum for these herbs is 5 percent apple cider vinegar, ensuring adequate acidity.

The Deer Tick Bite Prophylactic Formula

HERB	PLANT PART	WEIGHT TO VOLUME	MENSTRUUM PROPORTIONS
Cryptolepis sanguinolenta	Dried root	1:5 (or possibly 1:7; see the instructions in part 1 on page 103)	60% alcohol, 35% spring water, 5% apple cider vinegar
Houttuynia cordata	Fresh aerial parts (preferred)	1:2	65% alcohol, 35% spring water
	Dried aerial parts (if that's all that is available)	1:5	
Polygonum cuspidatum	Fresh root	1:3	50% alcohol, 50% spring water
	Dried root	1:5	60% alcohol, 40% spring water
Uncaria tomentosa	Dry bark	1:5	60% alcohol, 35% spring water, 5% apple cider vinegar

NOTES ON TINCTURING

× 100 grams of dried herb equals approximately 3.5 ounces; 150 grams fresh herb equals about 5.25 ounces.

× With dried herbs, you will lose 30 to 40 percent of the volume of the menstruum used to tincture, even if you strain and press carefully. Fresh herbs, though, will give you 100-plus percent of the volume of the menstruum you used; the moisture from the fresh plant matter will add to the total volume of liquid.

× These instructions will give you approximately 1,200 mL (1.25 quarts or 40 ounces), which will provide full-dosage treatment for approximately 2.5 months.

PART 1: TINCTURE THE DRIED HERBS

Dried herbs are frequently tinctured in a 1:5 ratio of herb weight to menstruum volume. Houttuynia is best tinctured from fresh plant material (see part 2 on page 105), but if you must use dried houttuynia, follow the procedure described here. For our purposes, tincture each herb separately.

1 Grind the dried herb to a moderately coarse powder. Using a scale, measure out 100 grams of the dried ground herb and put it into a widemouthed quart jar with a tight-fitting lid. (Since cryptolepis is very hard, you may need a Vitamix or comparably sturdy blender to grind it. If you can't achieve a moderately coarse powder of cryptolepis with your blender, you'll end up with a larger volume and may need more liquid than is called for in order to cover it; you could increase the herb-to-menstruum ratio from 1:5 to 1:7.)

2 Prepare the menstruum using the appropriate proportions of alcohol, spring water, and apple cider vinegar:

- ✗ *CRYPTOLEPIS SANGUINOLENTA*: 60% alcohol, 35% spring water, and 5% apple cider vinegar. For a total of 500 mL, combine 300 mL of alcohol with 175 mL of water and 25 mL apple cider vinegar.

- ✗ *HOUTTUYNIA CORDATA*: 65% alcohol and 35% spring water. For a total of 500 mL, combine 325 mL of alcohol with 175 mL of water.

- ✗ *POLYGONUM CUSPIDATUM*: 60% alcohol and 40% spring water. For a total of 500 mL, combine 300 mL of alcohol with 200 mL of water.

- ✗ *UNCARIA TOMENTOSA*: 60% alcohol, 35% spring water, and 5% apple cider vinegar. For a total of 500 mL, combine 300 mL of alcohol with 175 mL of water and 25 mL of apple cider vinegar.

3 Pour the menstruum over the dried herb powder and stir until all of the powder is wet. Seal the jar with its lid.

4 Set the jar in a spot at room temperature and out of direct light. Let steep for 21 days, shaking vigorously frequently.

5 Thoroughly wet and then wring out the T-shirt or polyester material.

6 Strain out the powdered herb by pouring the tincture through the wet T-shirt or polyester material into a fresh jar. Wearing rubber gloves (both because alcohol is drying to the skin and to keep the tincture clean), wring out any liquid you can from the remaining wet pulp, adding it to the tincture in the jar.

PART 2: TINCTURE THE FRESH HERBS

For tincturing fresh herb matter, we use a 1:2 or 1:3 ratio of plant weight to menstruum volume.

1 Chop the fresh herb into small pieces. (If you're using knotweed root, you may need to use clippers to chop it into small chunks.) Using a scale, measure out the chopped fresh herb and put it into a blender. For houttuynia, we use a 1:2 ratio of plant weight to menstruum volume, so you would need 150 grams of the herb. For Japanese knotweed, we use a 1:3 ratio, so you would need 100 grams.

2 Prepare the menstruum using the appropriate proportions of alcohol and spring water:

  × *HOUTTUYNIA CORDATA*: 65% alcohol and 35% spring water. For a total of 300 mL, combine 195 mL of alcohol with 105 mL of water.

  × *POLYGONUM CUSPIDATUM*: 50% alcohol and 50% spring water. For a total of 300 ml, combine 150 ml of alcohol with 150 ml of water.

3 Add the menstruum to the chopped fresh herb in the blender. Blend until mashed.

4 Transfer the contents of the blender to a clean jar. Seal the jar with its lid.

5 Set the jar in a spot at room temperature and out of direct light. Let steep for 21 days, shaking vigorously frequently.

6 Thoroughly wet and then wring out the T-shirt or polyester material.

7 Strain out the plant matter by pouring the tincture through the wet T-shirt or polyester material into a fresh jar. Wearing rubber gloves (both because alcohol is drying to the skin and to keep the tincure clean), wring out any liquid you can from the remaining wet pulp, adding it to the tincture in the jar.

PART 3: COMBINE THE TINCTURES IN THE APPROPRIATE RATIOS

See the formulas earlier in this chapter for the appropriate tincture ratios. For the deer tick formula, you'll combine *Cryptolepis sanguinolenta*, *Houttuynia cordata*, *Polygonum cuspidatum*, and *Uncaria tomentosa* tinctures in a 1:1:1:1 ratio — that is, in equal parts. (Though if you have slightly more or less of one or two herb tinctures, it will not change the overall efficacy of your extract.)

1 Add 60 mL of each tincture to a 240 mL bottle (that's about 8 ounces total).

2 Label the bottle with the name of the formula it contains. Store in a cool, dark spot, where the tincture will keep for up to 3 years.

3 Use the tincture according to the directions for deer tick bite prophylaxis described earlier in this chapter.

Key Herbs and an Enzyme: Profiles

LET'S TAKE A LOOK AT THE HERBS USED in the prevention and treatment of acute tick-borne illness in more detail, particularly those used in the tick bite formulas and to treat acute Lyme disease. Each plant has numerous constituents that work together in various ways to allow your immune system to better kill tick-borne pathogens. For this reason, I recommend the use of whole herbs, not isolated constituents extracted from herbs.

Each plant has numerous constituents that work together in various ways to allow your immune system to better kill tick-borne pathogens.

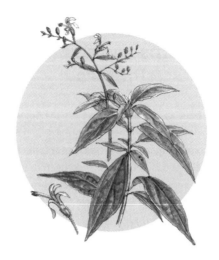

Andrographis paniculata

COMMON NAME: Andrographis

Andrographis is an extremely bitter herb that has been used for two thousand years in the traditional herbal medicine of India.

Andrographis kills *Borrelia* species and is used for the treatment of acute Lyme disease. It has potent anti-inflammatory effects and inhibits the inflammatory cytokines that become activated with Lyme disease. It improves macrophage and neutrophil activity. It protects the heart, improves liver function, and protects the liver. Because it can cross the blood-brain barrier, it kills *Borrelia* in the brain and protects neural and glial cells. Andrographis also relieves joint inflammation and swelling, prevents cartilage destruction, and has antiviral action.

Because it kills *Borrelia* species, andrographis is also useful as prophylaxis for *Ornithodoros* tick bites; *Borrelia* is the only pathogen these ticks are known to carry.

Like most plants, andrographis contains many active constituents. Andrographilides is the most popular and most researched constituent, and therefore you will often find a standardized extract of 10 percent andrographilides. However, since all constituents in the plant are beneficial, I recommend using the whole plant.

SIDE EFFECTS AND CONTRAINDICATIONS

The main side effects that may occur from using andrographis are possible gastrointestinal discomfort, constipation, dizziness, palpitations, or skin reactions. A rare side effect is a temporary loss of taste. Do not use if you are pregnant, if you are trying to become pregnant, or if you have active gall bladder disease. Do not use if you are taking isoniazid, theophylline, or immunosuppressants (e.g., cyclosporin). A very small percentage of people are allergic to andrographis. An allergic reaction would manifest as hives (an itchy skin rash); swelling of the mouth, lips, tongue, or throat; or wheezing or difficulty breathing. If you experience an allergic reaction, discontinue using the herb, and consider using diphenhydramine (Benadryl) or seeking medical attention.

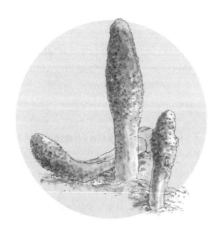

Cordyceps militaris, C. sinensis

COMMON NAME: Cordyceps

The common name *cordyceps* applies to two species that can be used interchangeably in the tick bite formulas and tick-borne disease treatments: *Cordyceps sinensis*, a brown-orange fungus native to higher altitudes of Asia, and *C. militaris*, a species more commonly known as orange caterpillar fungus.

Cordyceps has been used for thousands of years in the traditional medicinal practices of Tibet. It protects the liver, brain, and heart, has antibacterial and antiviral properties, and has adaptogen-like effects on the immune system and mitochondrial activity. Cordyceps is specifically effective as a cytokine modulator in *Rickettsia* treatment. It is also rich in amino acids, fatty acids, minerals, and vitamins.

SIDE EFFECTS AND CONTRAINDICATIONS

Cordyceps occasionally causes dry mouth or gastrointestinal discomfort. It has a synergistic effect with cyclosporin A and antidiabetic medications.

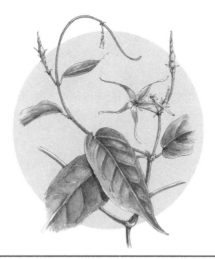

Cryptolepis sanguinolenta

COMMON NAME: Cryptolepis

Cryptolepis is a broad-spectrum antimicrobial herb used in the prophylaxis and treatment of babesiosis. A climbing perennial with thin stems, cryptolepis has been used for hundreds of years in Africa for the treatment of malaria and for thousands of years in Asia for various ailments.

Cryptolepis is immune modulating, anti-inflammatory, analgesic, fever reducing, and protective to the heart and the liver. It also has antiviral action and is incredibly effective against malaria. One study showed that mice given cryptolepis before being infected with malaria were protected against the disease.[46] I offer the extrapolation of this principle in support of using cryptolepis for the prevention of babesiosis with the herb's inclusion in the deer tick bite formula (page 91).

SIDE EFFECTS AND CONTRAINDICATIONS

The only noted side effect is a possible elevation in alkaline phosphatase and uric acid that resolves upon discontinuation with no adverse effect. These side effects have no clinical significance.

KEY HERBS AND AN ENZYME: PROFILES

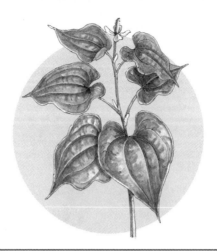

Houttuynia cordata

COMMON NAME: Houttuynia

Houttuynia is an invasive rhizomatous perennial that grows as ground cover in moist areas. It is an antimicrobial herb used to target *Anaplasma*, Powassan virus, and *Ehrlichia* in the deer tick bite formula, and it can also be used to target *Rickettsia*, *Bartonella*, Heartland virus, and Colorado tick fever virus.

Houttuynia has been shown to increase anti-inflammatory cytokines and decrease inflammatory cytokines in the immune system. As herbalist Stephen Buhner writes, houttuynia "inhibits viral replication, interferes with the function of the viral envelope, is directly virucidal, stops virion release from infected cells, and prevents viral infection if taken prophylactically."[47] As a result, houttuynia is included in tick bite formulas targeted at ticks that carry Powassan virus, Heartland virus, and Colorado tick fever virus. Houttuynia also has analgesic, antifungal, and antioxidant characteristics.

SIDE EFFECTS AND CONTRAINDICATIONS

The main side effect that may occur with houttuynia is nausea due to the herb's fishy smell and taste. Do not take during pregnancy.

Finding Fresh Houttuynia

Houttuynia is best used fresh. You can grow it in your garden, but fair warning: it spreads quickly and is difficult to eradicate, and in some regions it's considered an invasive species. You might consider growing it in pots. Or just look around your neighborhood — anyone who has a stand of it in their yard might be happy to let you dig some up. Avoid the variegated variety, which is less medicinally active.

Herbalist Bonnie Bloom, who makes the tinctures I use with patients, has a large garden of *houttuynia* plants. She is happy to sell plants inexpensively to people willing to pick them up at her farm site in Greenfield, Massachusetts. Find her company, Blue Crow Botanicals, in the Resources.

You can also order fresh houttuynia plants to be shipped to you from Strictly Medicinal Seeds (see Resources). Note that they have it listed under the common name "chameleon plant."

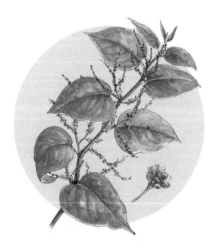

Polygonum cuspidatum

COMMON NAME: Japanese Knotweed

Japanese knotweed is another significantly important herb used to treat borreliosis and specifically Lyme disease. It is a leafy, bamboo-like perennial plant that grows and spreads easily. Japanese knotweed has been used as medicine in Asia for thousands of years. It is an invasive species in the United States, since it has been difficult to eradicate since its introduction in the early 1800s; in fact, some states now prohibit the live plant from being distributed or cultivated within their borders. Root harvesting is best done in spring or fall, although the process is challenging due to its deep root system and ease of sprouting.

Japanese knotweed counteracts the effect *Borrelia* has on the immune system. Knotweed blocks the cytokine-stimulated inflammatory response that is triggered by *Borrelia*, which weakens *Borrelia*'s effect on us and strengthens our immune system's effort to eradicate it. It has an anti-inflammatory effect on the joints and protects the heart. Japanese knotweed is very effective in treating neurological manifestations of Lyme disease, since it crosses the blood-brain barrier. Therefore, it is able to act as an antibacterial, anti-inflammatory, and antioxidant and has a calming effect in the brain and central nervous system. Japanese knotweed also protects endothelial cells that line blood vessels, creates blood vessel growth, and increases blood flow to the eyes, heart, skin, and joints. The plant has been shown to be a mild biofilm buster, decreasing the formation of biofilm and the amount of bacteria inside the biofilm. It also has antifungal and antiviral properties. In addition to treating Lyme disease, Japanese knotweed kills *Bartonella* species.

At least 67 constituents have been identified in Japanese knotweed. Resveratrol, which is abundant in this plant, is the most researched and widely used. Resveratrol is an antioxidant that improves neuromuscular coordination, learning, and memory; it protects the mitochondria and increases cerebral blood flow and oxygen to the brain. It also reduces inflammation (including joint inflammation) and protects cartilage. Red wine is another source of resveratrol. For the purposes of borreliosis prevention and treatment, I recommend using the whole herb instead of resveratrol alone. As noted above, the whole herb is generally preferable to an isolated constituent, and there are many other known chemical compounds found in knotweed that are effective against borreliosis. For example, like resveratrol, the polydactin, emodin, stillbenes, and anthraquinones in Japanese knotweed have a neuroprotective effect. Polydactin also protects the heart.

SIDE EFFECTS AND CONTRAINDICATIONS

The main side effect from using Japanese knotweed is possible gastrointestinal discomfort. A rare side effect is a temporary loss of taste. Do not use if you are pregnant, if you are trying to become pregnant, while taking anticoagulants, or before surgery.

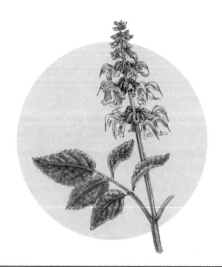

Salvia miltiorrhiza

COMMON NAME: Red Sage

Red sage, also known as dan shen, is a perennial shrub with dark green leaves and whorls of purple-blue flowers that is native to China and Japan. It has been used in Chinese medicine for over two thousand years. Like Chinese skullcap, red sage has potent adaptogen-like activity for cytokines, meaning that if the cytokine activity is high, it will lower it, and when cytokine activity is too low, it will raise it, according to what is best for the human body. This is especially helpful when the immune system is faced with an infection.

Red sage is especially effective as a cytokine modulator in *Rickettsia* treatment. (It inhibits COX-2, interleukin-17, and prostaglandin E, in this way working against the effects by which *Rickettsia* takes over the immune and endothelial systems.) It protects endothelial cells and gut mucosa as well as mitochondria, the spleen, the liver, and the heart. It also protects the Golgi apparatus (an organelle involved in intracellular transport, among other things), especially in brain cells, which can help prevent neurodegenerative disease.

SIDE EFFECTS AND CONTRAINDICATIONS

Red sage is an anticoagulant and should not be used with anticoagulant medications, if you have a bleeding disorder, or before surgery. It also inhibits the CYP3A4, CYP2C9, CYP2E1, CYP2D6, and CYP1A2 enzymes found in the liver, which are essential for the metabolism of certain medications. Since the herb inhibits these enzymes, this means that less medication is broken down and therefore more medication remains in the system. There is a long list of medications, called CYP3A4 substrates, that are affected by red sage, including acetaminophen, some antibiotics, statin drugs, many psychiatric drugs, opioids, some chemotherapeutic drugs, and immunosuppressants. CYP2C9, CYP2E1, CYP2D6, and CYP1A2 substrates are also affected by red sage. In rare cases, red sage can stimulate an allergic reaction. Do not use if you are pregnant.

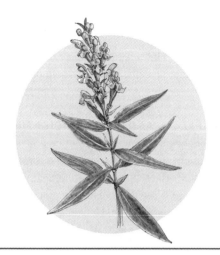

Scutellaria baicalensis

COMMON NAME: Chinese Skullcap

Chinese skullcap — not to be confused with American skullcap (*Scutellaria lateriflora*) — is a shrub with blue-purple helmet-shaped flowers that grows in sandy, moist areas. It is native to East Asia.

The root of Chinese skullcap has antibacterial, antiviral, and antifungal properties. It has an affinity for the brain, where it reduces inflammation, acts as an anticonvulsant, regulates sleep, stimulates brain tissue regeneration, and protects the neurological system. It blocks the pro-inflammatory cytokines that have been implicated in tick-borne diseases and protects the mitochondria.

Chinese skullcap has adaptogen-like effects on cytokine activity in *Rickettsia* treatment. As a way of survival, *Rickettsia* interacts with the human immune system to keep the level of several cytokines low enough that the bacteria can survive but high enough to keep its host alive. Chinese skullcap modulates the immune system in favor of the human body. If cytokine activity is high, it will lower it, and when cytokine activity is too low, it will raise it. (In particular, Chinese skullcap inhibits COX-2, p38 MAP kinase, and prostaglandin E2 and downregulates interleukin-17.) These actions work against *Rickettsia* as it tries to take over the immune and endothelial systems. Chinese skullcap is also effective in the treatment of Lyme disease.

SIDE EFFECTS AND CONTRAINDICATIONS

Chinese skullcap can sometimes cause gastrointestinal discomfort. It also inhibits the CYP3A4 enzyme found in the liver, which is essential for the metabolism of certain medications. Since the herb inhibits the enzyme, less medication is broken down and therefore more medication remains in the system. There is a long list of medications called CYP3A4 substrates that are affected by Chinese skullcap, including acetaminophen, some antibiotics, statin drugs, many psychiatric drugs, opioids, some chemotherapeutic drugs, and immunosuppressants. One of Chinese skullcap's constituents, oroxylin A, improves the efficacy of certain anticancer drugs by inhibiting the P-glycoprotein-mediated efflux pump. Chinese skullcap also increases the effect of ribavirin, albendazole, ciprofloxacin, and amphotericin B. Do not use if you are pregnant.

Serrapeptase

Serrapeptase, or serratiopeptidase, is an enzyme that was isolated from the bacterium *Serratia* that lives in the intestine of the silkworm. It has anti-inflammatory and anticoagulant properties. Most important, it has the ability to break down the matrix of biofilm that *Borrelia* and other tick-borne pathogens create around themselves. In conjunction with other pharmaceutical and/or herbal antibiotic strategies, a biofilm buster like serrapeptase is of utmost importance in eradicating the disease. It has been shown to be synergistic with some antibiotics.

SIDE EFFECTS AND CONTRAINDICATIONS

Because serrapeptase is an anticoagulant, do not take it before surgery, with anticoagulant medications, or if you have a bleeding disorder.

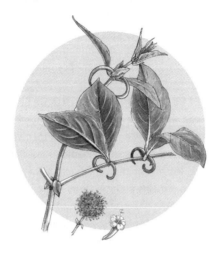

Uncaria rhynchophylla, U. tomentosa

COMMON NAME: Cat's Claw

Cat's claw, or *uña de gato*, is a woody vine with clawlike thorns. It is one of the most important herbs used to treat *Borrelia* infections, especially Lyme disease.

There are two species of *Uncaria* used in the treatment of Lyme disease. *Uncaria tomentosa* is well known and well researched. It is the species indicated in the tick bite formulas for prophylaxis of borreliosis. It is especially effective in preventing Lyme disease from taking hold in the body due to its effect on the immune system. Therefore, it is a key herb to use in prophylaxis. *U. tomentosa* is also effective as an anti-inflammatory in the joints, which may be painful or swollen in acute Lyme disease, as well as persistent Lyme disease (which is not covered in the scope of this book). Antiviral and antioxidant are other actions of *U. tomentosa* that are relevant to its use in preventing and treating acute tick-borne disease. It has been used by people living in the Amazon for thousands of years.

U. rhynchophylla is used to treat acute Lyme disease as well as persistent Lyme disease. *U. rhynchophylla* is especially effective when *Borrelia* has penetrated the blood-brain barrier. It has an anti-inflammatory and antiseizure effect on the brain, and is considered an excellent protector of the neurological system. Studies have shown that it works in numerous ways specifically in the brain: decreasing swelling, improving memory, improving learning, decreasing inflammation, protecting neurons, decreasing seizures, improving demyelination, increasing microglia (the connective tissue of the brain), and moderating aggression. Other relevant actions of *U. rhynchophylla* are that it is an antiviral and systemic tonic. It has been used in China for thousands of years.

U. tomentosa contains pentacyclic oxindole alkaloids (POA) and tetracyclic oxidize alkaloids (TOA); they are main constituents of the plant. Although *U. rhynchophylla* has some of these alkaloids, they are in the bark of the root and not the inner bark of the vine, which is the part of the plant used to treat Lyme disease. TOAs are especially effective in treating neurological effects of Lyme disease, while POAs improve immune function. There is some discussion around whether TOAs reduce the effect of POAs. Herbalist and Lyme authority Stephen Buhner does not support this claim. There are many products available, like Samento, that are TOA-free. In my experience, the traditional extraction process of *U. tomentosa* that includes both TOAs and POAs does not seem more or less effective than a TOA-free product.

SIDE EFFECTS AND CONTRAINDICATIONS

The main side effect from using *Uncaria* is possible gastrointestinal discomfort. *U. rhynchophylla* is a hypotensive, and therefore should be used with caution if you are on antihypertensive medication. Do not use if you are pregnant, if you are trying to become pregnant, while taking anticoagulants, if you are undergoing an organ transplant, before surgery, or while you are taking immunosuppressive drugs (e.g., cyclosporin).

CHAPTER 5

After a Tick Bite: What to Do

Ticks are small! Humans are most at risk for receiving tick bites from nymph (second life stage) and adult (third life stage) ticks. Remember, nymph deer ticks are the size of a poppy seed, whereas an adult is the size of a sesame seed.

In this chapter, we'll talk about what you can do to protect yourself from tick-borne diseases when a tick has bitten you.

1. Immediately remove and identify the tick.
2. Apply first aid.
3. Have the tick tested for pathogens.
4. Begin the herbal prophylactic protocol.
5. Watch for symptoms.
6. Get tested (maybe).

Attachment

A tick may take minutes to hours to choose the location for attachment and to start feeding. When a hard tick, like the blacklegged deer tick, attaches to a host, it secretes an adhesive cement-like compound over the first 5 to 30 minutes that secures the tick in place and makes it more difficult to detach. Once attached to a host, larvae and nymphs grow up to 20 times their original size, while adults grow up to 200 times their size.

Not all ticks are infected with or transmit pathogens. The time it takes to transmit a pathogen from a tick to a host depends on the species of tick, the pathogen titer (concentration), duration of feeding time, and the extent of tissue infection at the time of blood feeding. Some pathogens like *Borrelia burgdorferi*, *Anaplasma*, *Rickettsia rickettsii*, and *Babesia* must undergo a period of replication and/or expansion before transmission.

A review of studies on pathogen transmission and attachment times shows that it takes from 4 to 72 hours for an attached deer tick to transmit *Borrelia burgdorferi*.[48] Studies examined mice, deer, and humans as hosts. It took 24 to 50 hours for *Anaplasma* to transmit to mice and 36 hours to 18 days to transmit *Babesia* to hamsters and voles. *Borrelia mayonii* and *B. miyamotoi* took 24 to 96 hours to transmit to mice. Viruses, which are less common, need little to no replication and/or expansion time. For example, transmission time for Powassan virus is a short 15 to 30 minutes.

Ticks that have been attached to a host for a short period of time, allowing for them to partially feed, will attach to another host to complete their blood meal. One study showed that partially fed nymphal ticks detach from mice 15 percent of the time, and that 10 percent of questing nymphal ticks are distended from a partial blood meal.[49] These partially fed ticks that attach to a second host have a shorter pathogen transmission time. Within 24 hours, 83 to

100 percent of partially fed nymphal deer ticks had transmitted *Borrelia burgdorferi* to mice, and within 48 hours 100 percent of partially fed nymphal deer ticks had transmitted *B. burgdorferi* to mice.[50] Similar studies looking at humans as the host are needed. Ultimately, the longer the tick is attached, the higher the likelihood of transmission. Furthermore, it has been shown that people tend to underestimate the actual time the tick was attached in studies that compared tick engorgement to the subjective estimate of tick attachment.[51]

A Tick Preparedness Kit

× Tick Twister by O'Tom (there are other tools for removing ticks, but this one is my favorite and, in my experience, the most effective)

× Small ziplock bag (for collecting the tick)

× Andrographis tincture with dropper

× Homeopathic *Ledum palustre* 30C

× Homeopathic *Apis mellifica* 30C

× Tick bite prophylactic formula(s) specific to the types of ticks in your region

Immediately Remove and Identify the Tick

YOUR FIRST ACTION SHOULD BE TO REMOVE THE TICK quickly and without agitating it. Do not use a match, alcohol, petroleum jelly, or soap to encourage the tick to "back out" of the skin, as the tick may regurgitate pathogens as it does so. It is important to remove the mouthparts of the tick. The mouthparts include an anchoring organ, called a rostrum, that is covered with backward-curving hooks, which makes it difficult to remove the entire tick in a nondisruptive way with tweezers. The best approach is to use a tick-twisting system. The Tick Twister by O'Tom is an excellent option. If you only have tweezers within reach, grasp the tick as close to the skin as possible and pull upward.

If the mouthparts separate from the tick's body and remain embedded in your skin, often it's best to leave them there rather than trying to dig them out to avoid infection from any pathogens on the surface of the surrounding skin.

Once the tick is removed, place it in a plastic ziplock bag. Identify it (refer to chapter 1 and the Tick ID card at the end of this book) so that you can determine which pathogens may have been transmitted. Mark the date of the tick bite on your calendar.

TICK TWISTING TOOL:

1. Slide the twister over the tick from the side, so that the tick is held in the groove between the two tines of the tool.

2. Rotate the twister and tick, pulling upward just very gently.

3. At about five rotations, the tick should lift free.

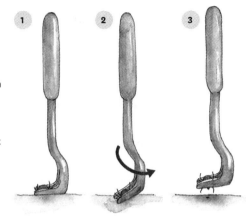

TWEEZERS:

1. Grasp the tick as close to the skin as possible.

2. Pull straight upward.

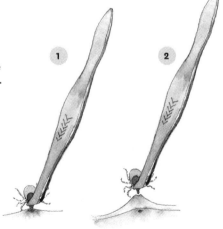

STEP 2
Apply First Aid
••••••••••••••••••••••••••

IF YOU WERE BITTEN BY A DEER TICK, put andrographis tincture over the area of the bite wound. Andrographis will kill *Borrelia* in the feces that were released by the tick onto the skin and that may be dragged into the wound by touching it. If you do not have andrographis available, use cat's claw or Japanese knotweed. Better yet, put deer tick bite formula (page 91) over the bite wound to address all the possible pathogens carried by the deer tick.

If you received a bite from a tick other than a deer tick, use the tick bite formula designed for the tick you removed. If you do not have any of those options available, use an over-the-counter antiseptic like rubbing alcohol or antibacterial cream like Neosporin.

Homeopathy offers another effective first-aid measure for a tick bite. Homeopathic medicine is based on the law of similars, or "like cures like" — a substance that would normally cause specific symptoms if taken by a healthy person would actually heal those symptoms in a sick person. A common example is taking onion, or *Allium* since the Latin is used in this system, for allergies. Whereas an onion would normally cause watery eyes and a runny nose in a healthy person, the homeopathic remedy of onion (*Allium*) is used to treat those symptoms of allergies. In the homeopathic remedy, the substance itself is very diluted. The law of infinitesimals addresses this concept, where it is held that the lower the dose of the medicine, the more potent the treatment. Homeopathy may be used as a complement to, but not in place of, proper medical assessment and treatment.

Ledum palustre 30C is a homeopathic remedy that may be taken after a tick bite to encourage healing. It is suggested to take three pellets under the tongue three times daily for 3 days.

Apis mellifica 30C is a homeopathic remedy that may be taken if the tick bite causes a rash, feels hot to the touch, or looks red. It is suggested to take three pellets under the tongue three times daily for 3 days.

STEP 3
Have the Tick Tested for Pathogens
∙∙∙∙∙∙∙∙∙∙∙∙∙∙∙∙∙∙∙∙∙∙∙∙

IF YOU GET A TICK BITE, I recommend that you send the tick to a laboratory to be tested to determine which pathogens it may be carrying. Among the variety of companies to choose from, I recommend TickReport. Since 2006, this facility, housed at the University of Massachusetts at Amherst Laboratory of Medical Zoology, has developed ways to test for a variety of pathogens and continues to expand its database of ticks from around the country. It uses highly specific, highly sensitive qPCR testing that detects the DNA of pathogens in the tick. At the time of this writing, TickReport can test for *Anaplasma phagocytophilum*, *Babesia divergens*, *B. duncani*, *B. microti*, *Bartonella henselae*, *Borrelia* species (and also specifically *Borrelia burgdorferi* sensu lato, *Borrelia lonestari*, *Borrelia miyamotoi*, and *Borrelia mayonii*), *Ehrlichia canis*, *E. chaffeensis*, *E. ewingii*, *E. muris*–like agent (aka *E. muris eauclairensis*), *Francisella tularensis*, *Rickettsia parkeri*, *R. philipii*, *R. rickettsii*, Bourbon virus, Colorado tick fever virus, Heartland virus, and Powassan virus.

When you send a tick to TickReport for testing, the lab identifies the type of tick, notes whether the tick had started feeding, and then tests for a range of pathogens, depending on the level of testing you ask for. The lab keeps ticks on file indefinitely so that a customer may request testing for other pathogens at a later date. See the Resources for contact information.

Without waiting for the tick testing results, you'll begin step 4, the herbal prophylactic protocol, taking the formula appropriate to the tick that bit you.

STEP 4
Begin the Herbal
Prophylactic Protocol

COMMON APPROACHES TO THE TREATMENT of a tick bite include watching and waiting for signs and symptoms, taking a single dose of doxycycline, or taking a longer course of antibiotics such as doxycycline, amoxicillin, cefuroxime, or azithromycin.[52] While these antibiotics kill the spirochete form of *Borrelia*, and doxycycline also kills *Anaplasma*, *Ehrlichia*, and *Rickettsia*, these antibiotics do not kill the round body form of *Borrelia*, *Babesia*, or viruses or break through the biofilm that is most likely surrounding some of these pathogens.

A better protocol, in my opinion, is this: After you receive a tick bite, immediately start a course of the appropriate prophylactic formula. I don't recommend waiting for symptoms to occur or blood testing to be completed before initiating this treatment. Which formula you use depends upon the type of tick that bit you, as we discussed in chapter 4.

For example, prophylactic treatment of deer tick bites would include treatment for borreliosis, anaplasmosis, babesiosis, ehrlichiosis, and Powassan virus because those are the diseases caused by the pathogens potentially carried by the deer tick. Therefore, I recommend treating every deer tick bite, whether or not symptoms have developed, according to the following principles:

× Activate the immune system to function better in the face of tickborne pathogens.

- × Target the free spirochete form of *Borrelia burgdorferi* and other *Borrelia* species.
- × Target the round body form of *B. burgdorferi*.
- × Target *Anaplasma*.
- × Target *Babesia*.
- × Target *Ehrlichia muris eauclairensis*.
- × Target Powassan virus.
- × Target biofilm.
- × Protect the joints, neurological system, heart, eyes, and liver.

The deer tick bite formula on page 91 does all this.

If you received a tick bite, did not get the tick tested for pathogens, and are asymptomatic, take the tick bite formula appropriate for the type of tick that bit you, following the dosage recommendations outlined with the formulas in chapter 4. Be sure to include the serra-peptase. Follow that protocol for 1 month.

If you received a tick bite and the tick tested negative for patho-gens, no further action is needed. You can stop taking the prophylactic formula.

If you received a tick bite, the tick tested positive for pathogens, and you are asymptomatic, begin treatment using herbs that are specific to the diseases caused by the pathogens found in the tick because those are the pathogens that may have been transmitted to you through the tick bite. Add serrapeptase as well. Chapter 6 provides a list of formulas per disease. *Remember that a tick testing positive for a pathogen does not mean that the pathogen was trans-mitted to you.*

If you received a tick bite and develop symptoms, review the test-ing options described in Step 6 and the treatment options described in chapter 6, and be sure to consult with your health-care provider.

STEP 5
Watch for Symptoms

∙∙∙∙∙∙∙∙∙∙∙∙∙∙∙∙∙∙∙∙∙∙∙∙∙∙∙∙∙∙∙∙∙∙∙∙∙

ONCE YOU START THE TICK BITE TREATMENT, begin watching for symptoms. If the tick that bit you tested positive for pathogens, watch for symptoms of the specific diseases caused by those pathogens. Mark the day you received the tick bite on your calendar to help you remember how many days it has been since the bite. This will be important information to have if you develop symptoms.

As we've discussed, symptoms vary depending on the type of tick-borne disease. See chapter 2 for details. They usually become evident within 30 days but can take up to several months (as in the case of Lyme disease and babesiosis) to manifest.

Symptoms can include the following:

- Rash
- Fever
- Flu-like symptoms
- Lymph nodes swelling
- Joint pain and/or swelling
- Muscle pain
- Tingling or numbness
- Bell's or facial palsy (drooping of one or both sides of the face)
- Headaches
- Sensitivity to light
- Neck pain or stiffness
- Nausea, vomiting, abdominal pain, loss of appetite
- Diarrhea
- Confusion, disorientation
- Cough
- Palpitations
- Night sweats
- "Air hunger" or nonexertional shortness of breath
- Chest pain
- Sore throat
- Drowsiness
- Difficulty speaking
- Hearing loss
- Loss of coordination
- Seizures
- Lethargy
- Paralysis

Rashes

It is normal for a tick bite to cause local irritation, most often in a circular area with a diameter of up to 1 centimeter. It can be helpful to measure the diameter of your rash and even draw a line around the perimeter of the rash. Then you can watch it to see if it expands.

A Lyme rash (erythema migrans) is diagnosed when a rash surrounding a tick bite reaches a diameter of more than 5 centimeters. It can be pink to red in color, may or may not feel warm to touch, may or may not be circular with central clearing (bull's-eye), and may be flat or raised. It usually spreads in a centrifugal fashion from around the bite outward. It may be more difficult to see on darker-skinned individuals. (Take a look at the Lyme rash ID guide in the back of this book for some examples.) If you have found a rash surrounding a tick bite on your body that fits the description, take a picture of it and go to your health-care provider, the emergency room, or an urgent care center to have it diagnosed, documented, and treated. Then see the section on the treatment of acute tick-borne disease in chapter 6.

Rocky Mountain spotted fever can cause a full-body rash that starts 2 to 6 days after the onset of fever, with a flat pink rash on the ankles, wrists, or forearms that spreads to the palms, soles, arms, legs, and trunk, usually sparing the face. It may create petechiae — clusters of tiny, flat, circular spots on the surface of the skin caused by bleeding under the skin. It may also become a raised pink, red, or purple rash. Most people with Rocky Mountain spotted fever have a rash at some point in their illness (and thus the name of the disease!).

People with anaplasmosis may also show signs of a rash, though it's relatively rare (affecting less than 10 percent of patients), while up to one-third of people with erhlichiosis experience a rash. In either case, it usually presents as a pinpoint or splotchy rash, typically not itchy and sparing the face, palms, and soles. In ehrlichiosis, the rash usually occurs 5 days after the fever, and it is more common with infection by *E. chaffeensis* and in children.

Normal Rash

- ✕ Local irritation at the site of the tick bite
- ✕ Circular in shape
- ✕ Up to 1 centimeter in diameter

Abnormal Rash (Possibly a Sign of Disease)

- ✕ More than 5 centimeters in diameter at the site of the tick bite
- ✕ Follows a fever
- ✕ Appears on other parts of the body (e.g., hands, feet, arms, ankles), away from the site of the tick bite
- ✕ Petechiae
- ✕ Eschar or ulcer at the site of the tick bite

Report Symptoms!

If you experience any symptoms of tick-borne disease after a tick bite, report them to your medical practitioner. Depending on your practitioner's level of literacy in the diagnosis and treatment of Lyme and other tick-borne diseases, consider consulting a Lyme-literate practitioner (see page 180).

STEP 6
Get Tested (Maybe)
·································

THERE ARE TWO SPECIFIC SITUATIONS in which you might consider getting tested for tick-borne disease: if the tick that bit you tests positive for specific pathogens, or if you develop symptoms. This is not in place of but in addition to treating the tick bite prophylactically.

If TBD testing seems appropriate, contact your health-care provider to discuss your options. The details can be complicated. Some pathogens are easier to test for than others. For some (like *Borrelia burgdorferi*), we have many options when it comes to testing technology, with varying levels of accuracy; with others, our testing options are limited. Some tests can be run at a regular commercial lab; others are best sent to a specialty laboratory. If you are considering TBD testing, I outline my general recommendations in the chart on page 138. Use this information to inform the conversation with your health-care provider.

The Types of Tests

There are many different testing techniques available for *Borrelia burgdorferi* and other tick-borne pathogens. They can generally be divided into two categories: indirect and direst testing.

INDIRECT TESTING

Indirect tests look for human antibodies instead of the pathogen or genetic material from the pathogen. Antibodies are proteins made by the immune system when it comes into contact with a pathogen. Immunoglobulin M (IgM) and immunoglobulin G (IgG) are two types of antibodies that indirect tests commonly look for as evidence of an immune response to a pathogen.

DIRECT AGGLUTINATION (DA): a technique used to detect antibodies to a particular pathogen. Antibodies from the human blood sample react with the antigen of the pathogen to make an antigen-antibody complex that clumps together (agglutinates).

INDIRECT IMMUNOFLUORESCENCE ANTIBODY (IFA) ASSAY: a technique used to detect antibodies (IgM and IgG) to a particular pathogen. Pathogen-specific antigens are used to bind to human antibodies in a human blood sample. Then secondary antibodies against human antibodies are added, which bind to the human antibodies. The secondary antibodies are bound to fluorescent labels.

ELISA (ENZYME-LINKED IMMUNOSORBENT ASSAY): a technique used to detect pathogen-specific antibodies. Pathogen-specific antigens are used to bind to human antibodies in a human blood sample. Then secondary antibodies against human antibodies are added, which bind to the human antibodies. The secondary antibodies are bound to an enzyme. In the last step, a colored substrate is added, which binds with the enzymes and displays color (indicating a positive reaction).

WESTERN BLOT: a technique used to detect pathogen-specific antibodies (IgM and IgG). It provides qualitative data regarding which specific antibodies are present in a human blood sample. It is more accurate than IFA and ELISA testing. Basically, a Western blot is an ELISA plus additional technology. Gel electrophoresis is used in order to separate human antibodies based on molecular weight, and the colored substrate added in the end will present with colored bands.

IMMUNOBLOT: a technique used to detect pathogen-specific antibodies (IgM and IgG). It provides qualitative data regarding which specific antibodies are present in a human blood sample. It is more accurate than IFA, ELISA, and Western blot testing. Basically, an immunoblot is a Western blot that utilizes technology that places pathogen-specific antigens on a membrane used in the electrophoresis.

DIRECT TESTING

Direct tests look for evidence of the pathogen by looking for the pathogen itself or genetic material of the pathogen.

WRIGHT-GIEMSA STAINED PERIPHERAL BLOOD SMEAR: a technique that identifies a pathogen by using a series of stains placed over a drop of blood that is smeared onto a slide. The stains allow you to clearly differentiate a pathogen like *Babesia* merozoites (stained purple) in the form of a ring or a "maltese cross" inside a red blood cell (stained pink). It is only reliable if the amount of pathogens in the blood is high enough, which only happens very early during an infection.

POLYMERASE CHAIN REACTION (PCR): a technique that identifies the DNA or RNA of a pathogen in the blood. It is best done early in a disease process, while there is still genetic material in the bloodstream. It lacks accuracy, especially later in the disease process, because it tests for genetic material only in the blood, while most of it will be in tissues. For example, the DNA of *B. burgdorferi* is only detected in early Lyme disease in 18 to 26 percent of blood samples.[53]

FLUORESCENCE IN SITU HYBRIDIZATION (FISH): a technique that identifies the DNA or RNA of a pathogen in the blood. Starting with a blood smear, a probe of short DNA or RNA molecule with a fluorescent label is added. The fluorescent probe binds to the pathogen's DNA or RNA, flagging the pathogen. FISH technology is much more accurate than the Giemsa stain for identifying a pathogen in red blood cells.

CULTURE: In the near future, specialty labs will be able to identify *Borrelia* itself from a blood culture.

Recommended Tests for
Tick-Borne Pathogens

PATHOGEN	DISEASE	TESTS
Anaplasma phagocytophilum	Anaplasmosis	*A. phagocytophilum* PCR during the first week of illness; after that time, IFA assay for *A. phagocytophilum* IgM and IgG
Babesia spp.	Babesiosis	IGeneX *Babesia* FISH (note that the IFA assay for *Babesia* spp. IgM and IgG at regular commercial laboratories is less accurate)
Bartonella spp.	Bartonellosis	IGeneX *Bartonella* FISH (note that the IFA assay for *Bartonella henselae* IgM and IgG at regular commercial laboratories is less accurate)
Borrelia burgdorferi	Lyme disease	Lyme Western blot, IGeneX Lyme Western blot, or IGeneX Lyme ImmunoBlot
Borrelia hermsii	Tick-borne relapsing fever	Wright-Giemsa stained peripheral blood smear; IGeneX TBRF ImmunoBlot
Borrelia mayonii	Lyme disease	IGeneX Lyme ImmunoBlot
Borrelia miyamotoi	Tick-borne relapsing fever	IGeneX TBRF ImmunoBlot
Borrelia parkeri	Tick-borne relapsing fever	Wright-Giemsa stained peripheral blood smear; IGeneX TBRF ImmunoBlot
Borrelia turicatae	Tick-borne relapsing fever	Wright-Giemsa stained peripheral blood smear; IGeneX TBRF ImmunoBlot
Colorado tick fever virus	Colorado tick fever	IFA assay for Colorado tick fever IgM and IgG
Ehrlichia chaffeensis	Ehrlichiosis	*Ehrlichia chaffeensis* PCR during the first week of illness; after that time, IFA assay for *E. chaffeensis* IgM and IgG

PATHOGEN	DISEASE	TESTS
Ehrlichia ewingii	Ehrlichiosis	Mayo Clinic *Ehrlichia* PCR; after that time there is no specific test, but due to antibody cross-reactivity, the IFA assay for *Ehrlichia chaffeensis* IgM and IgG may detect this pathogen as well
Ehrlichia muris eauclairensis	Ehrlichiosis	Mayo Clinic *Ehrlichia* PCR during the first week of illness; after that time there is no specific test, but due to antibody cross-reactivity, the IFA assay for *Ehrlichia chaffeensis* IgM and IgG may detect this pathogen as well
Francisella tularensis	Tularemia	Direct agglutination test for *Francisella tularensis* antibody
Heartland virus	Heartland virus	Heartland virus PCR by Medical Diagnostic Laboratories
Powassan virus	Powassan virus	Powassan virus PCR or Powassan virus IgG/IgM by ELISA by Medical Diagnostic Laboratories
Rickettsia parkeri	Rickettsiosis	*R. parkeri* PCR by Medical Diagnostic Laboratories
Rickettsia philipii	Rickettsiosis	*Rickettsia philipii* PCR by Medical Diagnostic Laboratories
Rickettsia rickettsii	Rickettsiosis	IFA assay for *R. rickettsii* IgM and IgG
Unknown	Southern tick-associated rash illness	No testing is available

NOTE: Some of the tests listed here are proprietary to IGeneX and Medical Diagnostic Laboratories, both of which offer high-quality testing for tick-borne diseases. You can find contact information for both labs in the Resources of this book. If a specific lab is not indicated, any commercial lab is sufficient.

SNAPSHOT:
Tick-Borne Pathogens

If you decide to get tested to determine whether you've been exposed to a particular tick-borne disease, the pathogens you test for will be determined by the tick that bit you (which is why tick identification is so important!). Here's a list of the pathogens that may be present in each type of tick.

Blacklegged Tick/Deer Tick (*Ixodes scapularis*)

Anaplasma phagocytophilum
Babesia species
Borrelia burgdorferi
Borrelia mayonii
Borrelia miyamotoi
Ehrlichia muris eauclairensis
Powassan virus

Western Blacklegged Tick/Deer Tick (*Ixodes pacificus*)

Anaplasma phagocytophilum
Babesia duncani
Borrelia burgdorferi
Borrelia miyamotoi

American Dog Tick (*Dermacentor variabilis*)

Francisella tularensis
Rickettsia rickettsii

Lone Star Tick (*Amblyomma americanum*)

Ehrlichia chaffeensis
E. ewingii
Francisella tularensis
Heartland virus
STARI

Brown Dog Tick (*Rhipicephalus sanguineus*)

Rickettsia rickettsii

Gulf Coast Tick (*Amblyomma maculatum*)

Ehrlichia chaffeensis
Rickettsia parkeri

Rocky Mountain Wood Tick (*Dermacentor andersoni*)

Colorado tick fever virus
Francisella tularensis
Rickettsia rickettsii

Ornithodoros Ticks

Borrelia hermsii
Borrelia parkeri
Borrelia turicatae

CASE STUDY:
Testing after a Deer Tick Bite

After an *Ixodes scapularis* or *I. pacificus* deer tick bite, it is appropriate to consider testing for *Borrelia burgdorferi* (Lyme disease), *B. miyamotoi* (tick-borne relapsing fever), *Anaplasma*, *Babesia*, and Powassan virus. If you received a tick bite in the north-central United States, consider also testing for *Ehrlichia muris eauclairensis* and *B. mayonii* (Lyme disease).

Testing for Lyme disease in a human is not recommended until 4 weeks after the tick bite since antibodies may not be produced by the immune system until that point. Lyme disease testing looks for the immune system's response to coming into contact with *Borrelia* and making antibodies. The currently available Lyme testing tells you not whether you currently have Lyme disease but, rather, whether you have ever been exposed to it.

Let's review the testing options for Lyme disease from lowest accuracy to highest accuracy. Extensive research shows that, unfortunately, the ELISA, the conventional standard test, is not reliable.[54] The ELISA test is set up as a two-tiered test: if the ELISA is negative, the Western blot is not done; if the ELISA is positive, the Western blot is done. But skipping the ELISA and directly running a Lyme disease Western blot IgM and IgG through a regular commercial laboratory is a better option than the ELISA because it is more sensitive (more accurate). I usually recommend testing by IGeneX, a private company that uses a highly sensitive Lyme disease Western blot IgM and IgG that is prepared from strains B31 and 297 and looks for additional specific antibodies. While a regular commercial laboratory usually uses just *B. burgdorferi* strain B31, IGeneX also uses strain 297. In my opinion, an IGeneX Western blot test is a better option than a Western blot from a commercial lab. However, the Western blot test does not detect all of the *B. burgdorferi* sensu lato antibodies. Therefore, the very best option at the time of this writing is the newer IGeneX Lyme ImmunoBlot IgM and IgG test, which detects the widest range of antibodies that I'm aware of, including antibodies to *B. burgdorferi* strains B31 and 297 as well as *B. afzelii*, *B. garinii*, *B. mayonii*, *B. spielmanii*, and *B. californiensis*. Available since 2018, this IGeneX test provides a sensitivity of 90.9 percent.[55]

Next, depending on your location, it may be appropriate to consider testing for *B. miyamotoi*, a bacterium that causes tick-borne relapsing fever (TBRF). The PCR testing for *B. miyamotoi* that is typically done at a regular commercial laboratory is accurate only if done within the first 3 days of illness. I recommend instead the IGeneX TBRF ImmunoBlot.

If you have had a deer tick bite, it is also appropriate to test for anaplasmosis and babesiosis. Conventional testing for anaplasmosis at a regular commercial laboratory is sufficient. If you are testing during the first week of illness, use the PCR amplification test for

Anaplasma phagocytophilum. If you are testing after the first week of illness, an IFA assay for *A. phagocytophilum* IgM and IgG is best.

I do not recommend testing for babesiosis at a regular commercial lab, since the standard IFA assay for *Babesia microti* IgM and IgG is not reliable. Instead, I recommend using the IGeneX FISH assay to test for all *Babesia* species. It is a highly sensitive and specific test that detects ribosomal RNA with a blood smear.

Depending on your location, you may consider testing for Powassan virus, though it is still a rare tick-borne disease as of this writing. I recommend Powassan virus testing by PCR or IgG/IgM by ELISA by Medical Diagnostic Laboratories.

After an *Ixodes* tick bite in the north-central United States, it is appropriate to consider testing for *Ehrlichia muris eauclairensis*. For *Ehrlichia muris eauclairensis*, you can use PCR amplification testing during the first week of illness; after that time there is no specific test, but due to antibody cross-reactivity, the IFA assay for *Ehrlichia chaffeensis* IgM and IgG may detect this pathogen as well.

Be aware that testing may be less reliable in special populations, including immunocompromised people (who may not be able to mount an adequate immune response) and pregnant women (whose hormonal changes may affect immune response).

. . .

Please consult a Lyme-literate medical practitioner to discuss and order appropriate testing after a tick bite. See chapter 6 for more details.

Acute Tick-Borne Disease Treatment

When a disease is diagnosed soon after a tick bite, this is considered to be the acute stage. This chapter reviews treatment strategies for acute tick-borne disease. We'll build on the signs and symptoms discussed in chapter 2 and look at specific protocols used to treat each disease. These protocols often include pharmaceutical antibiotics as well as herbal antimicrobials. The good news is, prompt comprehensive treatment of acute tick-borne disease usually results in full recovery.

What to Do If You
Develop Symptoms

IF YOU DEVELOP SYMPTOMS AFTER A TICK BITE, i call this a symptomatic tick bite. The treatment of a symptomatic tick bite is different from the treatment of an asymptomatic bite — that is, one that does not produce symptoms of disease. With symptoms surfacing, there is a possible active infection. Therefore, report symptoms to a medical professional, preferably someone who is Lyme and TBD literate. If such a provider is not available, visit your health-care provider, the emergency room, or an urgent care center.

If you think you have found a bull's-eye rash on your body or rash around a tick bite that is increasing in size, take a picture of the rash. Then take a pen or marker, draw a line around the edge of the rash, measure the rash's diameter, and jot that measurement down. As its name *migrans* suggests, an erythema migrans, or the Lyme rash, will migrate or spread outward from the bite site on the body. It will over time grow to a diameter of at least 5 centimeters. Give your health-care provider a description of this kind of a rash along with any other symptoms you may be experiencing. Ultimately, an erythema migrans is diagnostic for Lyme disease. Therefore, the treatment of an erythema migrans rash is a treatment for active, current Lyme disease (see next section). A blood test is not needed to confirm Lyme disease in the case of a diagnosed erythema migrans. In the absence of an erythema migrans, but with the development of other new symptoms, diagnosis is more complicated and blood tests may be appropriate.

If you have not already started a tick bite formula appropriate for the tick that bit you (refer to chapter 4), I recommend starting the formula immediately after noticing symptoms. See chapter 4 for dosages. The tick bite formulas should be taken on an empty stomach — that is, 30 minutes before food and 2 hours after food. Also, I recommend using the biofilm buster serrapeptase (see page 119) at 500 mg or 120,000 units twice daily on an empty stomach.

Depending on the constellation of symptoms after a tick bite, I might recommend a specific treatment that includes pharmaceutical antimicrobials in addition to using a tick bite formula and serrapeptase. No matter what protocol you follow, I recommend continuing treatment for 2 months past the resolution of symptoms in order to eradicate the disease.

Beginning Treatment for Acute Tick-Borne Disease

IF YOU ARE DIAGNOSED WITH ACUTE LYME or other tick-borne disease, that means you have a current active infection that must be treated. I recommend finding a Lyme-literate practitioner to work with. Once symptoms appear or a disease has been diagnosed, shift gears from prevention to active treatment of disease. Pharmaceutical antimicrobials are most effective when used immediately upon diagnosis. In addition, the appropriate herbal antimicrobials and serrapeptase may be used with any of the protocols. The more tools used in the beginning of treatment, the less likely there will be an ongoing infection, especially with Lyme disease.

In this section, we'll examine acute tick-borne disease treatment plans that use both pharmaceutical and herbal antimicrobials. Since no two cases of Lyme or any other tick-borne disease are alike, treatment should be individualized to each person. Although there are basic principles to follow when treating TBD, I find it crucial to customize the treatment. Many factors like age, drug allergies, alcohol use, sun exposure, side effects, history of antibiotic use, and history of gastrointestinal disease/distress are considered in creating the optimal plan. And it bears reiterating: it is important to continue treatment for 2 months past the point when symptoms resolve.

All of the treatments in this chapter are designed for an average 150-pound nonpregnant adult. For information on adjusting the dosages for children, see page 98. For information on treating tick-borne disease in pregnancy, see page 160.

Acute Lyme Disease Treatment

In the event of an erythema migrans, diagnosed Lyme disease, or the development of symptoms after a tick bite that indicate Lyme disease, a specific treatment approach is indicated, one that treats all the ways Lyme bacteria exist and hide in the body. The spirochete form of the *Borrelia* can be treated by certain pharmaceutical and herbal antibiotics. The most common antibiotic used to treat Lyme disease is doxycycline. Other pharmaceutical antibiotics that can kill the spirochete form are cefuroxime, amoxicillin, azithromycin, clarithromycin, and trimethoprim-sulfamethoxazole. To eradicate the infection, however, it's important to add additional treatment. The round body form of the bacterium can be treated by only a select few pharmaceutical antibiotics like metronidazole, tinidazole, and hydroxychloroquine. Adding the following herbal antibiotics to address the round body form is recommended: cat's claw, Japanese knotweed, and andrographis. Grapefruit seed extract also kills the round body form. All of the herbal antibiotics used to treat Lyme disease have the ability to kill both the spirochete form and the round body form.

In addition, the issue of biofilm must be tackled. As we discussed in chapter 2, biofilm is a shell that pathogens create around themselves to survive. Pharmaceutical antibiotics are not effective against biofilm. A treatment protocol must utilize a natural biofilm buster like serrapeptase, nattokinase, lumbrokinase, bromelain, oregano oil,

N-acetyl-cysteine, or stevia to break through biofilm. Then the bacteria that are hiding inside biofilm will be exposed to the pharmaceutical and/or herbal antibiotics. Addressing the ways in which *Borrelia* hides will create a more effective treatment. I emphasize, again, the importance of treating the infection for 2 months after symptoms have resolved. Stopping treatment too soon is a common mistake and often leads to the return of symptoms.

Here is a typical acute Lyme disease treatment protocol that I recommend for a nonpregnant adult (and children with the adjustment of dosage based on weight):

1. **DOXYCYCLINE:** Two 100 mg capsules twice a day, with breakfast and dinner. Avoid products with high levels of calcium, magnesium, or iron (for example, dairy products, almond products, and antacids) within 2 hours before or after. Avoid the sun while taking doxycycline due to the increased risk of photosensitivity.

   If doxycycline cannot be used, or if photosensitivity is of great concern (as may be the case in summer), cefuroxime (500 mg twice daily) or azithromycin (500 mg once daily) are appropriate alternatives.

2. **LYME/BORRELIOSIS FORMULA I:** Combine equal parts of *Uncaria tomentosa* inner vine bark tincture, *Uncaria rhynchophylla* inner vine bark tincture, *Polygonum cuspidatum* root tincture, and *Andrographis paniculata* aerial parts tincture; take 1 teaspoon in water three times a day, 30 minutes before breakfast, lunch, and dinner.

3. **LYME/BORRELIOSIS FORMULA II (OPTIONAL):** Combine equal parts of *Polygonum cuspidatum* root tincture, *Pueraria lobata* root tincture, *Salvia miltiorrhiza* root tincture, and *Scutellaria baicalensis* root tincture; take 1 teaspoon in water three times a day, 30 minutes before breakfast, lunch, and dinner.

4. **SERRAPEPTASE:** 500 mg or 120,000 units twice a day, 30 minutes before breakfast and dinner.

5. **PROBIOTICS:** 40 billion organisms daily, 2 hours before or after antibiotics.

The second Lyme/borreliosis formula in this protocol is optional but helpful. It contains a combination of herbs that preserves the body's natural immune response to *Borrelia* and prevents the bacteria from steering the immune response in favor of their survival. It also offers significant neurological and joint support, bolstering two systems commonly affected by *Borrelia*.

Acute Anaplasmosis Treatment

Fortunately, anaplasmosis responds very well to treatment and does not tend to cause an ongoing infection. Doxycycline is the only antibiotic that treats *Anaplasma*, and it does so very well. The American Academy of Pediatrics Committee on Infectious Diseases recommends doxycycline in children of all ages as the first-line treatment of anaplasmosis.

Here is a typical acute anaplasmosis treatment protocol that I recommend for a nonpregnant adult (and children with the adjustment of dosage based on weight):

1. **DOXYCYCLINE:** Two 100 mg capsules twice a day, with breakfast and dinner. Avoid products with high levels of calcium, magnesium, or iron (for example, dairy products, almond products, and antacids) within 2 hours before or after. Avoid the sun while taking doxycycline due to the increased risk of photosensitivity.

2. **ANAPLASMOSIS/EHRLICHIOSIS FORMULA:** Combine 3 parts *Houttuynia cordata* aerial parts tincture, 3 parts *Salvia miltiorrhiza* root tincture, 2 parts *Astragalus membranaceus* root tincture, 2 parts *Pueraria lobata* root tincture, and 2 parts *Scutellaria*

baicalensis root tincture; take 1¼ teaspoons in water three times a day, 30 minutes before breakfast, lunch, and dinner.

3. **SERRAPEPTASE:** 500 mg or 120,000 units twice a day, 30 minutes before breakfast and dinner.

4. **PROBIOTICS:** 40 billion organisms daily, 2 hours before or after antibiotics.

Acute Babesiosis Treatment

Here is a typical acute babesiosis treatment protocol that I recommend for a nonpregnant adult (and children with the adjustment of dosage based on weight):

1. **ATOVAQUONE:** 750 mg twice a day, with breakfast and dinner. Take with fat. Do not take coenzyme Q10 (CoQ10) while taking atovaquone. *Caution:* Your medical practitioner should monitor your liver and kidney function if you use this medication.

2. **AZITHROMYCIN:** One 500 mg pill with breakfast.

3. **BABESIA FORMULA:** Combine equal parts of *Cryptolepis sanguinolenta* root tincture, *Sida acuta* leaf tincture, and *Bidens pilosa* leaf and flower tincture; take 1 teaspoon in water three times a day, 30 minutes before breakfast, lunch, and dinner.

4. **SALVIA MILTIORRHIZA ROOT TINCTURE:** ½ teaspoon in water three times a day, 30 minutes before breakfast, lunch, and dinner.

5. **SERRAPEPTASE:** 500 mg or 120,000 units twice a day, 30 minutes before breakfast and dinner.

6. **PROBIOTICS:** 40 billion organisms daily, 2 hours before or after antibiotics.

Acute Ehrlichiosis Treatment

Fortunately, ehrlichiosis responds very well to treatment and does not tend to cause an ongoing infection. Doxycycline is the only antibiotic that treats *Ehrlichia*, and it does so very well. The American Academy of Pediatrics Committee on Infectious Diseases recommends doxycycline for children of all ages as the first-line treatment of ehrlichiosis.

Here is a typical acute ehrlichiosis treatment protocol that I recommend for a nonpregnant adult (and children with the adjustment of dosage based on weight):

1. **DOXYCYCLINE:** Two 100 mg capsules twice a day, with breakfast and dinner. Avoid products with high levels of calcium, magnesium, or iron (for example, dairy products, almond products, and antacids) within 2 hours before or after. Avoid the sun while taking doxycycline due to the increased risk of photosensitivity.

2. **ANAPLASMOSIS/EHRLICHIOSIS FORMULA:** Combine 3 parts *Houttuynia cordata* aerial parts tincture, 3 parts *Salvia miltiorrhiza* root tincture, 2 parts *Astragalus membranaceus* root tincture, 2 parts *Pueraria lobata* root tincture, and and 2 parts *Scutellaria baicalensis* root tincture; take 1¼ teaspoons in water three times a day, 30 minutes before breakfast, lunch, and dinner.

3. **SERRAPEPTASE:** 500 mg or 120,000 units twice a day, 30 minutes before breakfast and dinner.

4. **PROBIOTICS:** 40 billion organisms daily, 2 hours before or after antibiotics.

Acute Rickettsial Spotted Fever Group Treatment

It is of utmost importance to immediately treat rickettsial spotted fever group. Rocky Mountain spotted fever can be life threatening and requires treatment with a tetracycline antibiotic, like doxycycline. The CDC and the American Academy of Pediatrics Committee on Infectious Diseases recommend doxycycline for children of all ages as the first-line treatment of rickettsial spotted fever group. The duration of treatment is at least 10 days.

Here is a typical acute rickettsial spotted fever group treatment protocol that I recommend for a nonpregnant adult (and children with the adjustment of dosage based on weight):

1. **DOXYCYCLINE:** Two 100 mg capsules twice a day, with breakfast and dinner. Avoid products with high levels of calcium, magnesium, or iron (for example, dairy products, almond products, and antacids) within 2 hours before or after. Avoid the sun while taking doxycycline due to the increased risk of photosensitivity.

2. ***POLYGONUM CUSPIDATUM* ROOT TINCTURE:** 1 tablespoon in water three times a day, 30 minutes before breakfast, lunch, and dinner.

3. ***SALVIA MILTIORRHIZA* ROOT TINCTURE:** 1 teaspoon in water three times a day, 30 minutes before breakfast, lunch, and dinner.

4. ***SCUTELLARIA BAICALENSIS* ROOT TINCTURE:** 1 teaspoon in water three times a day, 30 minutes before breakfast, lunch, and dinner.

5. ***CORDYCEPS MILITARIS* OR *C. SINENSIS* TINCTURE:** 1 teaspoon in water three times a day, 30 minutes before breakfast, lunch, and dinner.

6. **SERRAPEPTASE:** 500 mg or 120,000 units twice a day, 30 minutes before breakfast and dinner.

7. **PROBIOTICS:** 40 billion organisms daily, 2 hours before or after antibiotics.

Acute Tularemia Treatment

The treatment of acute tularemia depends upon the severity of the infection. I have not treated acute tularemia in my practice, but I have included standard medical treatment guidelines (the pharmaceutical antibiotics listed) in addition to my herbal recommendations.

Here is an example of an acute tularemia treatment protocol for a nonpregnant adult (and children with the adjustment of dosage based on weight):

FOR SEVERE ILLNESS

1. **STREPTOMYCIN,** intravenous or intramuscular: 10 mg/kg every 12 hours for 10 days.

2. **GENTAMICIN,** intravenous or intramuscular: 5 mg/kg per day, in three divided doses, for 10 days.

3. *CRYPTOLEPIS SANGUINOLENTA* **ROOT TINCTURE:** 1 teaspoon in water three times a day, 30 minutes before breakfast, lunch, and dinner.

4. **SERRAPEPTASE:** 500 mg or 120,000 units twice a day, 30 minutes before breakfast and dinner.

5. **PROBIOTICS:** 40 billion organisms daily, 2 hours before or after antibiotics.

FOR MODERATE TO MILD ILLNESS

1. **DOXYCYCLINE,** intravenous or oral: 200–400 mg per day for 21 days.

2. **CIPROFLOXACIN,** intravenous or oral: 750 mg twice a day for 14 days.

3. ***CRYPTOLEPIS SANGUINOLENTA* ROOT TINCTURE:** 1 teaspoon in water three times a day, 30 minutes before breakfast, lunch, and dinner.

4. **SERRAPEPTASE:** 500 mg or 120,000 units twice a day, 30 minutes before breakfast and dinner.

5. **PROBIOTICS:** 40 billion organisms daily, 2 hours before or after antibiotics.

Acute Powassan Virus Treatment

There is no pharmaceutical antiviral treatment for Powassan virus. Most patients are hospitalized and receive intravenous fluids, respiratory support, and medication to decrease brain swelling. I have not treated acute Powassan virus, but I recommend the following protocol, based on Stephen Buhner's book *Herbal Antivirals*, in addition to conventional medical care.

1. **TICK-BORNE ENCEPHALITIS FORMULA:** Combine equal parts of *Glycyrrhiza glabra* root tincture, *Houttuynia cordata* aerial parts tincture, *Isatis tinctoria* root tincture, and *Scutellaria baicalensis* root tincture; take 1 teaspoon in water three times a day, 30 minutes before breakfast, lunch, and dinner.

2. **POWASSAN FORMULA I:** Combine 2 parts *Cordyceps militaris* or *C. sinensis* tincture, 1 part *Astragalus membranaceus* root tincture, and 1 part *Rhodiola rosea* tincture; take 1 teaspoon in water six times daily.

3. **POWASSAN FORMULA II:** Combine equal parts of *Ceanothus americanus* tincture, *Polygonum cuspidatum* root tincture, and *Pueraria lobata* root tincture; take 1 teaspoon in water three times a day, 30 minutes before breakfast, lunch, and dinner.

4. **POLYGALA TENUIFOLIA TINCTURE:** 30 drops in water three times a day, 30 minutes before breakfast, lunch, and dinner.

5. **HERICIUM ERINACEUS TINCTURE:** 1 teaspoon in water three times a day, 30 minutes before breakfast, lunch, and dinner.

6. **POWASSAN FORMULA III:** Combine equal parts of *Angelica sinensis* root tincture and *Salvia miltiorrhiza* root tincture; take 1 teaspoon to 1 tablespoon up to 10 times daily.

7. **POWASSAN FORMULA IV:** Combine equal parts of *Chelidonium majus* whole-plant tincture, *Leonurus cardiaca* aerial parts tincture, and *Ligusticum wallichii* tincture; take 1 teaspoon in water three times a day, 30 minutes before breakfast, lunch, and dinner.

8. **SERRAPEPTASE:** 500 mg or 120,000 units twice a day, 30 minutes before breakfast and dinner.

Acute Heartland Virus Treatment

There is no pharmaceutical antiviral treatment for Heartland virus. I have not treated acute Heartland virus, but I recommend the following, based on Stephen Buhner's book *Herbal Antivirals*.

1. **TICK-BORNE ENCEPHALITIS FORMULA:** Combine equal parts of *Glycyrrhiza glabra* root tincture, *Houttuynia cordata* aerial parts tincture, *Isatis tinctoria* root tincture, and *Scutellaria baicalensis* root tincture; take 1 teaspoon in water three times a day, 30 minutes before breakfast, lunch, and dinner.

2. **SERRAPEPTASE:** 500 mg or 120,000 units twice a day, 30 minutes before breakfast and dinner.

Acute Tick-Borne Relapsing Fever Treatment

Here is typical acute TBRF treatment protocol that I recommend for a nonpregnant adult (and children with the adjustment of dosage based on weight):

1. **TETRACYCLINE:** One 500 mg capsule every 6 hours. Avoid products with high levels of calcium, magnesium, or iron (for example, dairy products, almond products, and antacids) within 2 hours before or after. Avoid the sun while taking tetracycline due to the increased risk of photosensitivity.

    If tetracycline cannot be used, use doxycycline (200 mg every 12 hours) or erythromycin (500 mg every 6 hours). Cefuroxime (500 mg twice daily) may be used in the treatment of *Borellia miyamotoi* or *B. turicatae*.

2. **LYME/BORRELIOSIS FORMULA I:** Combine equal parts of *Uncaria tomentosa* inner vine bark tincture, *Uncaria rhynchophylla* inner vine bark tincture, *Polygonum cuspidatum* root tincture, and *Andrographis paniculata* aerial parts tincture; take 1 teaspoon in water three times a day, 30 minutes before breakfast, lunch, and dinner.

3. **LYME/BORRELIOSIS FORMULA II (OPTIONAL):** Combine equal parts of *Polygonum cuspidatum* root tincture, *Pueraria lobata* root tincture, *Salvia miltiorrhiza* root tincture, and *Scutellaria baicalensis* root tincture; take 1 teaspoon in water three times a day, 30 minutes before breakfast, lunch, and dinner.

4. **SERRAPEPTASE:** 500 mg or 120,000 units twice a day, 30 minutes before breakfast and dinner.

5. **PROBIOTICS:** 40 billion organisms daily, 2 hours before or after antibiotics.

Acute Colorado Tick Fever Treatment

There is no pharmaceutical antiviral treatment for Colorado tick fever virus. I have not treated acute Colorado tick fever, but I recommend the following, based on Stephen Buhner's book *Herbal Antivirals*.

1. **TICK-BORNE ENCEPHALITIS FORMULA:** Combine equal parts of *Glycyrrhiza glabra* root tincture, *Houttuynia cordata* aerial parts tincture, *Isatis tinctoria* root tincture, and *Scutellaria baicalensis* root tincture; take 1 teaspoon in water three times a day, 30 minutes before breakfast, lunch, and dinner.

2. **SERRAPEPTASE:** 500 mg or 120,000 units twice a day, 30 minutes before breakfast and dinner.

Acute STARI Treatment

Southern tick-associated rash illness (STARI) is most likely caused by a *Borrelia* species. Therefore, the treatment is the same as for Lyme disease.

Here is a typical acute STARI treatment protocol that I recommend for a nonpregnant adult (and children with the adjustment of dosage based on weight):

1. **DOXYCYCLINE:** Two 100 mg capsules twice daily, with breakfast and dinner. Avoid products with high levels of calcium, magnesium, or iron (for example, dairy products, almond products, and antacids) within 2 hours before or after. Avoid the sun while taking doxycycline due to the increased risk of photosensitivity.

   If doxycycline cannot be used, or if photosensitivity is of great concern (as may be the case in summer), cefuroxime (500 mg twice daily) or azithromycin (500 mg once daily) are appropriate alternatives.

2. **LYME/BORRELIOSIS FORMULA I:** Combine equal parts of *Uncaria tomentosa* inner vine bark tincture, *Uncaria rhynchophylla* inner vine bark tincture, *Polygonum cuspidatum* root tincture, and *Andrographis paniculata* aerial parts tincture; take 1 teaspoon in water three times a day, 30 minutes before breakfast, lunch, and dinner.

3. **LYME/BORRELIOSIS FORMULA II (OPTIONAL):** Combine equal parts of *Polygonum cuspidatum* root tincture, *Pueraria lobata* root tincture, *Salvia miltiorrhiza* root tincture, and *Scutellaria baicalensis* root tincture; take 1 teaspoon in water three times a day, 30 minutes before breakfast, lunch, and dinner.

4. **SERRAPEPTASE:** 500 mg or 120,000 units twice a day, 30 minutes before breakfast and dinner.

5. **PROBIOTICS:** 40 billion organisms daily, 2 hours away from antibiotics.

Acute Bartonellosis Treatment

While it has not been proven whether *Bartonella* is transmitted by ticks to humans, I do see persistent bartonellosis in my practice. I suspect that *Bartonella* was transmitted by contact with fleas in many cases.

Here is a typical acute bartonellosis treatment protocol that I recommend for a nonpregnant adult (and children with the adjustment of dosage based on weight):

1. **RIFAMPIN:** One 300 mg pill twice a day, with breakfast and dinner. Note that rifampin may cause urine and tears to take on an orange-red color. *Caution:* Your medical practitioner should monitor your liver and kidney function if you use this medication.

2. **AZITHROMYCIN:** One 500 mg pill with breakfast.

Tick-Borne Diseases and Pregnancy

Acquiring a tick-borne disease while pregnant poses extra concern due to possible transmission of some tick-borne diseases to the fetus as well as some limitations to treatment. In Lyme disease treatment, there are pharmaceutical antibiotic alternatives to doxycycline that are safe for use in preganancy, like cefuroxime and azithromycin. However, for anaplasmosis, ehrlichiosis, and Rocky Mountain spotted fever, doxycycline is the best and perhaps the only effective treatment. The CDC states that the use of doxycycline during pregnancy is unlikely to cause substantial negative effect on the development of the fetus, although it is not without risk.[56]

Since many herbs and supplements have not been studied for safety in pregnancy, by default they are not recommended. Cat's claw (*Uncaria tomentosa*) is an essential herb for the treatment of tick-borne disease that is safe in pregnancy. Please note that it will interfere with conception, however. Astragalus (*Astragalus membranaceus*) is another effective herb that is safe during pregnancy. Serrapeptase and probiotics are safe to use in pregnancy.

FOR THE TREATMENT OF LYME DISEASE, TICK-BORNE RELAPSING FEVER, OR STARI IN PREGNANCY: In addition to the appropriate pharmaceutical treatment, serrapeptase, and probiotics, take ½ teaspoon of cat's claw inner vine bark tincture and ½ teaspoon of astragalus root tincture 30 minutes before breakfast, lunch, and dinner.

FOR THE TREATMENT OF ANAPLASMOSIS, EHRLICHIOSIS, AND ROCKY MOUNTAIN SPOTTED FEVER IN PREGNANCY: In addition to the appropriate pharmaceutical treatment, serrapeptase, and probiotics, take 1 teaspoon of astragalus root tincture 30 minutes before breakfast, lunch, and dinner.

Please discuss all pharmaceutical and natural treatments with your health care practitioner and OBGYN when undergoing TBD treatment during pregnancy. As an alternative to alcohol extracts, cat's claw and astragalus glycerites (if desired) are available from Woodland Essence (see Resources).

3. **BARTONELLA FORMULA:** Combine equal parts of *Alchornea cordifolia* leaf tincture, *Houttuynia cordata* aerial parts tincture, and *Polygonum cuspidatum* root tincture; take 1 teaspoon in water three times a day, 30 minutes before breakfast, lunch, and dinner.

4. **SERRAPEPTASE:** 500 mg or 120,000 units, 30 minutes before breakfast and dinner.

5. **PROBIOTICS:** 40 billion organisms daily, 2 hours before or after antibiotics.

Pharmaceutical Antimicrobials

THE FOLLOWING PHARMACEUTICAL ANTIMICROBIALS are included in the acute tick-borne disease protocols discussed in this chapter.

DOXYCYCLINE is from the tetracycline family, a bacteriostatic antibiotic that crosses the blood-brain barrier. *Bacteriostatic* means that the agent stops the bacteria from reproducing. Doxycycline inhibits bacterial protein synthesis by binding to the 30S subunit of the ribosome — the smaller subunit of a bacterium's ribosome — and thereby slowing cell growth. It should be avoided in pregnancy and while breastfeeding except when no other antibiotic options exist. Side effects include severe sun sensitivity and gastrointestinal discomfort. Foods that are rich in magnesium, calcium, or iron, such as dairy and almond products, as well as antacids, should be avoided within 2 hours before or after you've taken doxycycline, as they will decrease its efficacy.

CEFUROXIME is from the cephalosporin family, a bactericidal antibiotic that crosses the blood-brain barrier. *Bactericidal* means that the agent kills the bacteria. Cefuroxime inhibits cell wall growth, thereby killing the cell. It is safe to use in pregnancy, while breastfeeding, and in children.

AZITHROMYCIN is from the macrolide family, a bacteriostatic antibiotic that has a limited ability to cross the blood-brain barrier. Azithromycin inhibits bacterial protein synthesis by binding to the 50S subunit of the ribosome and thereby slowing cell growth. It is used with atovaquone to treat babesiosis, which is caused by a protozoan, not a bacterium. It is safe to use in pregnancy, while breastfeeding, and in children.

ATOVAQUONE is an antimalarial drug from the class of naphthoquinones. Atovaquone inhibits the mitochondrial electron transport chain, thereby slowing growth. It must be taken with a high amount of fat to be best absorbed. Do not take with CoQ10, which will interfere with the efficacy of atovaquone.

STREPTOMYCIN AND GENTAMICIN, from the aminoglycoside family, are bactericidal antibiotics that have limited ability to cross the blood-brain barrier. They create fissures in the outer membrane of the bacterium and inhibit bacterial protein synthesis by binding to a part of the 30S subunit of the ribosome.

CIPROFLOXACIN is from the fluoroquinolone family, a bactericidal antibiotic that crosses the blood-brain barrier. Ciprofloxacin prevents replication of bacterial DNA. One side effect to note is the potential for tendonitis or tendon rupture.

RIFAMPIN, from the rifamycin family, is a bactericidal antibiotic that crosses the blood-brain barrier. Rifampin inhibits bacterial RNA synthesis. A side effect includes orange-red discoloration of bodily fluids like urine and tears.

Common side effects of pharmaceutical antimicrobials include nausea, vomiting, loose stool, and abdominal pain. Specific antimicrobials may have other side effects.

Pharmaceutical antibiotics are indiscriminate in killing bacteria; they destroy not only disease-causing bacteria but also the beneficial bacteria that help our bodies maintain gut health. For this reason, it is recommended to take probiotics — a replenishment of beneficial bacteria — while on an antibiotic regimen. Probiotics should be taken at least 2 hours before or after an antibiotic dose. They can prevent the gastrointestinal side effects of pharmaceutical antibiotics as well as prevent and treat *C. diff* (*Clostridioides difficile*), a secondary bacterial infection that can accompany the use of some antibiotics and causes watery diarrhea. Taking probiotics that contain the "good yeast" *Saccharomyces boulardii* has been shown to prevent *C. diff*.[57]

In addition to probiotics, I usually prescribe nystatin, a pharmaceutical antifungal agent, when antibiotics are used for longer than 1 month in order to prevent vaginal or oral candidiasis (yeast overgrowth). When taking antibiotics for over 1 month, you may add two 500,000-unit tablets of nystatin twice daily with the antibiotic prescribed.

This is not a complete list of the antimicrobials used to treat Lyme and other tick-borne diseases. Please discuss side effects, drug interactions, and contraindications with your prescriber.

Diet is also very important. I recommend avoiding foods that feed Lyme and tick-borne disease: sugar, yeast, and alcohol. You might also consider an anti-inflammatory diet. Be sure to drink at least 2 to 3 liters of water daily during treatment.

Finding a Lyme–Literate Practitioner
· · · · · · · · · · · · · · · · · · · ·

THERE ARE TWO MEDICALLY RECOGNIZED STANDARDS of care in the medical community for the diagnosis and treatment of Lyme disease and tick-borne disease. Conventional medical practitioners most often follow the CDC or the Infectious Diseases Society of America (IDSA) guidelines. However, guidelines are also available from the International Lyme and Associated Diseases Society (ILADS), which, as this nonprofit medical society describes itself, is focused on advancing the standard of care for Lyme and other tick-borne diseases through research, education, and policy. ILADS guidelines recommend longer and more comprehensive treatment and recognize a wider variety of effective diagnostic tests and treatment methods. The ILADS guidelines, in fact, are currently the only guidelines in compliance with the Institute of Medicine's standard for rigorous evidence assessment tool called GRADE.[58]

As a practitioner, I follow the ILADS guidelines in addition to relying on my own clinical experience. Since I have sought out additional education in the diagnosis and treatment of Lyme and tick-borne disease, I am considered to be a Lyme-literate naturopathic doctor (LLND). There are other Lyme-literate health-care professionals, like Lyme-literate medical doctors (LLMD), nurse practitioners, physician's assistants, acupuncturists, Chinese medicine doctors, and psychologists. Often, like myself, Lyme-literate health professionals are ILADS members, have trained with an ILADS medical practitioner, and attend conferences for continuing education.

Lyme-literate practitioners, by definition, support the idea that Lyme can continue to cause illness in the body past the initial acute phase of diagnosis and treatment. Lyme-literate medical professionals will take a complete history of your illness, will review lab results that you have had, and might recommend more accurate testing

Within the Lyme-literate community . . . there has been a bridging of conventional medicine and natural therapies. Past the initial phase of Lyme disease, a holistic approach has been realized to hold incredible value and importance.

for Lyme and other tick-borne diseases. They might recommend a longer-term treatment protocol.

Years ago, long-term antibiotics were the main treatment strategy for Lyme and other tick-borne diseases. More recently, as research and decades of clinical practice have provided us with a better understanding of the disease process and treatment, conventionally trained medical providers have embraced, researched, and utilized many strategies beyond pharmaceutical antibiotics. And so, within the Lyme-literate community, and specifically the ILADS community, there has been a bridging of conventional medicine and natural therapies. Past the initial phase of Lyme disease, a holistic approach has been realized to hold incredible value and importance.

A Lyme-literate naturopathic doctor (LLND) has learned more about the diagnosis and treatment of Lyme and tick-borne disease based on scientific evidence beyond the scope of conventional medical guidelines while employing naturopathic philosophy, diagnostic testing, and treatments. Naturopathic physicians emphasize finding the cause and treating the whole person. This treatment philosophy is inherently well suited for patients with chronic disease in general, and Lyme and TBD in particular. Lyme literacy calls upon integrative, complementary, or holistic medicine to fully address the needs and concerns of this special population of patients. It requires a special lens to truly see what is going on for these patients and address the causes of their disease.

You can find a Lyme-literate practitioner through any of the following organizations:

× International Lyme and Associated Diseases Society
× Global Lyme Alliance
× LymeDisease.org

See the Resources for contact information for these organizations.

Looking Ahead

THANK YOU FOR CHOOSING TO EDUCATE YOURSELF about how to stay tick-free and prevent tick-borne disease. In this book, we began with a review of ticks in North America and how to identify them. We discussed the top tick-borne diseases and the symptoms they cause. You learned about reducing the tick population and preventing tick bites through multiple strategies. We discussed herbal prophylaxis with tick bite formulas appropriate for the type of ticks in your area as a daily preventive measure or an immediate treatment for a tick bite. You are even prepared to make the proper tick bite formula yourself. We covered what to do after a tick bite, including immediate herbal treatment; how to proceed if you develop symptoms after a tick bite; what to do if you are diagnosed with an acute tick-borne disease; and how to find a Lyme-literate practitioner. You now know about the many resources available to support you in your tick-free journey and for guidance if you develop tick-borne disease. My mission is to end tick-borne disease through prevention of tick bites. My hope is that you enjoy living tick-free and empower others to do the same.

We are continuously learning more about ticks and tick-borne disease. Unfortunately, new ticks and tick-borne diseases are being discovered all the time. More research about tick-control methods for the land will emerge, as will tick repellents for personal use. I look forward to seeing nootkatone becoming commercially available in the future and have confidence it will make a huge impact as an outdoor acaricide and a personal tick repellent. Other tick-control approaches currently being studied include botanical acaricides, genetic modification of ticks, robotic tick control devices, and rodent vaccinations. I encourage you to watch for the discovery of new types of ticks, diseases they carry, and how to protect yourself from them.

It heartens me to see more people becoming more educated about Lyme and TBD prevention. Public awareness, education, and research are increasing. Politically, there has been a significant recent development: the federal Tick-Borne Disease Working Group, which was created under the 21st Century Cures Act, brings together medical, scientific, and policy experts as well as patient representatives to discuss the current state of TBD in the United States and make recommendations to Congress on policy changes. I encourage you to read the working group's 2018 and other reports to Congress and to participate in the ongoing process that is open for public comment (see Resources). The 2018 report provides an extensive description of the public health challenges caused by tick-borne disease and specific recommendations to address those challenges. Some of the recommendations include research to gain a better understanding of ticks and tick-borne disease, to create technology to quickly identify new tick-borne diseases, and to create better testing, as well as the promotion of tick-borne disease awareness and prevention to the public and medical professionals. I am encouraged by the momentum the task force has brought to the areas of research, education, and national policy. This critical work is a symbol of the shifting consciousness around Lyme and TBD in this country. As we anticipate these advancements, it is our personal responsibility to take active steps in staying tick-free and avoiding tick-borne disease, and to empower others to do the same. May this book provide you with the tools you need for that journey.

ACKNOWLEDGMENTS

THIS BOOK WOULD NOT HAVE BEEN POSSIBLE without the first phone call from Carleen Madigan of Storey Publishing in the spring of 2018, asking if I would be interested in writing a book on the prevention of Lyme disease. I had no idea of the adventure to come! Thank you for encouraging me to follow my passion for educating the public in creating this book.

I have endless gratitude for Nancy Ringer, editor extraordinaire with brilliant insight and grace.

My sincere thanks to the editors, illustrators, designers, and everyone else at Storey Publishing. You are an absolutely gifted team!

I am indebted to my mentors and to the physicians and researchers who have gone before me: Alan MacDonald, MD; Joseph Burrascano, MD; Charles Ray Jones, MD; Kenneth Liegner, MD; Eva Sapi, PhD; Wayne Anderson, ND; Neil Nathan, MD; Thomas Moorcroft, DO; Julia Greenspan, ND; Samuel Shor, MD; Lee Cowden, MD; and many more. A special thanks to all of those who have played a role in creating and maintaining the International Lyme and Associated Diseases Society (ILADS). Thank you for fostering a thoughtful community of researchers and clinicians committed to understanding the constantly evolving landscape of diagnosis and treatment of tick-borne disease.

I am especially grateful to Richard Horowitz, MD, with whom I interned and from whom I have continued to learn ever since. Thank you for passionately and articulately sharing your experience. I would not be where I am today if it were not for you. You instilled in me the confidence to explore what it means to become part of the solution of the tick-borne disease epidemic and to serve those suffering with tick-borne disease.

A special thanks to my colleagues and all of the staff at Sojourns Community Health Clinic. Thank you for creating a truly healing place to work. Every day it is a privilege and an honor to enter the truly special healing space created by each and every one of you. I am grateful for all that I learn from my patients and colleagues. I am especially indebted to Linda Campbell, RN; Gaelen Ewald, RN; Brianna Schaefer, CMA; and Felicity Ladd, RN; without you my work would be impossible! And a special thanks to Linda Haltinner, DC, who encouraged me to educate the public on Lyme disease early on.

Deep gratitude to Bonnie Bloom. It has been an honor to collaborate with you on making the healing herbal formulas, like the deer tick bite formula, available to many. Thank you for your herbal wisdom and love of the healing plants!

I am especially grateful to Stephen Harrod Buhner. Thank you for your brilliance in sharing your wisdom and compiling research on so many healing plants that have had a profound impact on my patients' lives. Your books have been instrumental in forming my fundamental understanding of, and utilization of, herbal medicine in my clinical practice.

It is with deepest gratitude that I acknowledge Jeff Wulfman, MD; thank you for your support and guidance.

Many thanks as well to Robert Giguere and Jyotsna Shah, PhD, at IGeneX Inc., for reviewing part of the laboratory testing section of my manuscript.

A special thanks to local eateries that fueled many hours of my writing: Prime Roast in Keene, New Hampshire, Tulip Café in Brattleboro, Vermont, and Northampton Coffee in Northampton, Massachusetts. Each of you ties for the best homemade almond milk chai, in my book! And to the Monadnock Food Co-op: thank you for nourishing me during my writing process and for being a hub of local, high-quality food and products.

Thank you to my patients — you have been my greatest inspiration!

I want to thank Valerie Clifton from the bottom of my heart: with your unconditional love, you inspired me to love myself and to be present in the moment. Thank you also to Lisa Melodia and Brendan Moroney for your friendship and encouragement and for reading my very first draft of the manuscript.

My thanks to Sivananda Ashram: you are an oasis of love and inspiration that served to ground me during some of my writing process. And to all of the special beings and spiritual places that have nourished my spiritual practice — I am a better human being because of you.

Most importantly, thanks to my wife, Ruth, my original proofreader, gourmet chef, and most cherished partner on this life's journey. I have deep gratitude for your enthusiasm, patience, love, and support.

Ticks by State and Province

This chart shows which ticks have been found in which U.S. states and Canadian provinces as of the latest reports, which generally date from between 2017 and 2019. An X indicates that a tick species has been found in a particular state or province, but remember that tick ranges can vary widely across a state or province, and tick species that carry specific diseases in some regions do not carry those same diseases in other regions.

	Blacklegged Tick (Deer Tick)	Western Blacklegged Tick (Western Deer Tick)	American Dog Tick	Lone Star Tick	Brown Dog Tick	Gulf Coast Tick	Rocky Mountain Tick	Ornithodoros Tick	Asian Longhorned Tick
UNITED STATES									
ALABAMA	×		×	×	×	×			
ALASKA	×		×	×	×				
ARIZONA		×			×		×	×	
ARKANSAS	×		×	×	×	×			×
CALIFORNIA		×	×		×		×	×	
COLORADO					×		×	×	
CONNECTICUT	×		×	×	×				×
DELAWARE	×		×	×	×	×			×
FLORIDA	×		×	×	×	×		×	
GEORGIA	×		×	×	×	×			
HAWAII					×				
IDAHO			×		×		×	×	
ILLINOIS	×		×	×	×				
INDIANA	×		×	×	×				
IOWA	×		×	×	×				
KANSAS	×		×	×	×	×		×	
KENTUCKY	×		×	×	×	×			×
LOUISIANA	×		×	×	×	×			
MAINE	×		×	×	×				
MARYLAND	×		×	×	×	×			×
MASSACHUSETTS	×		×	×	×				
MICHIGAN	×		×	×	×				
MINNESOTA	×		×	×	×				
MISSISSIPPI	×		×	×	×	×			
MISSOURI	×		×	×	×	×			
MONTANA			×		×		×	×	

	BLACKLEGGED TICK (Deer Tick)	WESTERN BLACKLEGGED TICK (Western Deer Tick)	AMERICAN DOG TICK	LONE STAR TICK	BROWN DOG TICK	GULF COAST TICK	ROCKY MOUNTAIN TICK	ORNITHODOROS TICK	ASIAN LONGHORNED TICK
UNITED STATES									
NEBRASKA	×		×	×	×	×	×		
NEVADA		×			×		×	×	
NEW HAMPSHIRE	×		×	×	×				
NEW JERSEY	×		×	×	×				×
NEW MEXICO					×		×	×	
NEW YORK	×		×	×	×				×
NORTH CAROLINA	×		×	×	×	×			×
NORTH DAKOTA	×		×		×		×		
OHIO	×		×	×	×				
OKLAHOMA	×		×	×	×	×		×	
OREGON		×	×		×		×	×	
PENNSYLVANIA	×		×	×	×				×
RHODE ISLAND	×		×	×	×				
SOUTH CAROLINA	×		×	×	×	×			
SOUTH DAKOTA	×		×		×		×		
TENNESSEE	×		×	×	×	×			×
TEXAS	×		×	×	×	×		×	
UTAH		×			×		×	×	
VERMONT	×		×	×	×				
VIRGINIA	×		×	×	×	×			×
WASHINGTON		×	×		×		×	×	
WEST VIRGINIA	×		×	×	×				×
WISCONSIN	×		×	×	×				
WYOMING					×		×	×	
CANADA									
ALBERTA	×		×		×	×	×		
BRITISH COLUMBIA	×	×	×		×		×	×	
MANITOBA	×		×						
NEW BRUNSWICK	×		×	×	×				
NEWFOUNDLAND AND LABRADOR*	×		×	×	×				
NOVA SCOTIA	×		×	×	×				
ONTARIO	×		×	×					
PRINCE EDWARD ISLAND	×								
QUEBEC	×		×	×	×				
SASKATCHEWAN	×		×				×		

*Newfoundland and Labrador form a single province, but in actuality, in Labrador only the blacklegged tick (deer tick) has been found.

Tick-Borne Disease by State and Province

This chart shows which tick-borne diseases have been found in which U.S. states and Canadian provinces. This information was gleaned from reports originating with the U.S. Centers for Disease Control, the Canadian ministry of health, various state departments of health, and other reputable sources. The time span in which cases were reported differs by disease, depending on when official agencies began collecting case reports, and the relevant dates for the United States are noted in parentheses with each disease below.

	Lyme Disease (2007–2017)	Anaplasmosis (as of 2017)	Babesiosis (2011–2018)	Ehrlichiosis (as of 2017)	Spotted Fever Rickettsiosis* (2017)	Tularemia+ (2007–2017)	Powassan Virus (2009–2018)	Heartland Virus (as of Sept. 2018)	Tick-Borne Relapsing Fever (1990–2015)	Colorado Tick Fever (2002–2012)
UNITED STATES										
ALABAMA	x	x	x	x	x	x				
ALASKA	x	NN		NN	NN	x				
ARIZONA	x	x			x	x			x	x
ARKANSAS	x	x		x	x	x		x		
CALIFORNIA	x	x	x		x	x			x	x
COLORADO	x	NN		NN	x	x			x	x
CONNECTICUT	x	x	x	x	x	x	x			
DELAWARE	x	x	x	x	x	x				
FLORIDA	x	x		x	x	x				
GEORGIA	x	x	x	x	x			x		
HAWAII		NN		NN	NN					
IDAHO	x	NN		NN	x	x			x	x
ILLINOIS	x	x	x	x	x	x		x		
INDIANA	x	x	x	x	x	x	x	x		
IOWA	x	x	x	x	x	x				x
KANSAS	x	x		x	x	x		x	x	
KENTUCKY	x	x	x	x	x	x		x		
LOUISIANA	x		x	x	x	x				
MAINE	x	x	x	x	x		x			
MARYLAND	x	x	x	x	x	x				
MASSACHUSETTS	x	x	x	x	x	x	x			
MICHIGAN	x	x	x	x	x	x				
MINNESOTA	x	x	x	x	x	x	x			
MISSISSIPPI	x		x‡	x	x					
MISSOURI	x	x		x	x	x		x		x
MONTANA	x	x		x	x	x			x	x
NEBRASKA	x		x	x	x	x				x
NEVADA	x				x	x			x	
NEW HAMPSHIRE	x	x	x	x	x	x	x			
NEW JERSEY	x	x	x	x	x	x	x			
NEW MEXICO	x	NN		NN	x	x			x	x

	Lyme Disease (2007–2017)	Anaplasmosis (as of 2017)	Babesiosis (2011–2018)	Ehrlichiosis (as of 2017)	Spotted Fever Rickettsiosis* (2017)	Tularemia† (2007–2017)	Powassan Virus (2008–2017)	Heartland Virus (as of Sept. 2018)	Tick-Borne Relapsing Fever (1990–2015)	Colorado Tick Fever (2002–2012)
UNITED STATES										
NEW YORK	×	×	×	×	×	×	×			
NORTH CAROLINA	×	×		×	×	×	×	×		
NORTH DAKOTA	×	×	×	×	×	×	×			
OHIO	×	×	×	×	×	×				
OKLAHOMA	×	×		×	×	×		×	×	
OREGON	×	×	×	×	×	×			×	×
PENNSYLVANIA	×	×	×	×	×	×	×			×
RHODE ISLAND	×	×	×	×	×		×			
SOUTH CAROLINA	×		×	×	×	×				
SOUTH DAKOTA	×	×	×	×	×	×				
TENNESSEE	×	×	×	×	×	×		×		
TEXAS	×	×	×	×	×	×			×	
UTAH	×	×			×	×			×	×
VERMONT	×	×	×	×	×	×				
VIRGINIA	×	×	×	×	×	×	×			
WASHINGTON	×	×	×	×	×	×			×	×
WEST VIRGINIA	×	×		×	×	×				
WISCONSIN	×	×	×	×	×	×	×			
WYOMING	×				×	×			×	×
CANADA										
ALBERTA		×			×	×				×
BRITISH COLUMBIA	×				×	×			×	×
MANITOBA	×	×	×			×			×	
NEW BRUNSWICK	×					×	×			
NEWFOUNDLAND AND LABRADOR	×					×				
NOVA SCOTIA	×	×			×	×				
ONTARIO	×	×	×	×	×	×	×			×
PRINCE EDWARD ISLAND	×					×				
QUEBEC	×	×				×	×			
SASKATCHEWAN	×				×	×				

NN = not notifiable; the state does not require cases of this disease to be reported.

*Spotted fever rickettsiosis is the name for a group of rickettsial diseases that includes Rocky Mountain spotted fever, *Rickettsia parkeri* rickettsiosis, Pacific Coast tick fever, and rickettsial pox.

†In addition to being found in all Canadian provinces, tularemia has also been reported in the three Canadian territories: Northwest Territories, Nunavut, and Yukon.

‡The CDC offers a map of reported babesiosis cases for 2011–2014, as well as a data table for that same time span, and in the case of Mississippi, at the time of this writing, the map and the table do not agree. The conflict in data leaves us not knowing whether babesiosis has been reported in Mississippi.

GLOSSARY

ANAPLASMOSIS. A tick-borne disease caused by the bacterium *Anaplasma phagocytophilum*.

ARCARICIDE. A substance toxic to mites or ticks.

ARGASID (SOFT) TICK. A tick having a soft shell and lacking a dorsal shield. Males and females look the same, their mouthparts are not visible from above, they feed rapidly, and humans are incidental hosts.

ASYMPTOMATIC. Displaying no symptoms of disease.

BABESIOSIS. A tick-borne protozoan disease caused by *Babesia microti*, *B. divergens*, and *B. duncani*.

BARTONELLOSIS. A disease caused by *Bartonella* species bacteria.

BIOFILM. A protective shell that pathogens create around themselves to survive.

COLORADO TICK FEVER. A tick-borne viral disease.

CYTOKINE. An immune messenger cell.

DORSAL SHIELD. A hard (sclerotized) plate on the back of a tick that is used to identify the tick. Also called the scutum.

EHRLICHIOSIS. A bacterial tick-borne disease caused by *Ehrlichia chaffeensis*, *E. ewingii,* and *E. muris eauclairensis*.

ENDOTHELIAL CELLS. Cells that line the interior surface of blood vessels and lymphatic vessels.

ERYTHEMA MIGRANS. A pink or red rash surrounding the tick bite that may or may not feel warm to the touch, may or may not be circular with central clearing (that makes it look like a bull's-eye), may be flat or raised, and is at least 5 cm in diameter. It usually spreads in a centrifugal fashion from around the bite outward. There may also be multiple bull's-eye rashes all over the body (known as disseminated erythema migrans).

HEARTLAND VIRUS. A tick-borne viral disease.

IXODID (HARD) TICK. A tick having a hard shell and needing three blood meals to complete its life cycle.

LARVA. In a tick, the first life stage.

LIPOPROTEINS. Outer membrane surface proteins.

LYME DISEASE. A disease caused by *Borrelia* bacteria; in the United States, *B. burgdorferi* sensu stricto and *B. mayonii* cause Lyme disease.

LYME LITERATE. Referring to a health-care professional who has learned more about the diagnosis and treatment of Lyme and tick-borne disease based on scientific evidence beyond the scope of conventional medical guidelines, and who supports the idea that Lyme can continue to cause illness in the body past the initial acute phase of diagnosis and treatment.

MENSTRUUM. A liquid solvent that pulls active constituents from the plants soaking in it.

NATUROPATHIC MEDICINE. A branch of medicine based on the belief that the body has an innate ability to heal. Naturopathic physicians are educated and trained at 4-year naturopathic medical colleges that are accredited by the Council on Naturopathic Medical Education (CNME) and have passed professional board examinations administered by the North American Board of Naturopathic Examiners (NABNE) in order to become licensed.

NYMPH. In a tick, the second life stage.

PATHOGEN. A microorganism capable of causing disease.

POWASSAN VIRUS. A tick-borne viral disease.

PROPHYLACTIC. Preventive.

PROPHYLAXIS. A measure taken to prevent disease or the spread of disease.

Q FEVER. An illness caused by the bacterium *Coxiella burnetii*.

QUESTING. In a tick, the act of a tick holding on to something in its environment — a blade of grass, a bit of leaf litter, the fibers of a dog bed — with its third and/or fourth pair of legs while reaching out with its first two pairs of legs, waiting to grab hold of a passerby.

RICKETTSIAL SPOTTED FEVER GROUP. A tick-borne disease caused by an infection with *Rickettsia* bacteria.

RICKETTSIOSIS. A disease caused by *Rickettsia* bacteria.

SENSU LATO. "In the broad sense," which at the time of this writing includes 19 species of *Borrelia* bacteria, four of which are known to cause Lyme disease.

SENSU STRICTO. "In the narrow sense," which refers to the one species known to cause Lyme disease in North America: *B. burgdorferi*.

SERRAPEPTASE. An enzyme that can break down the biofilm that many tick-borne pathogens create around themselves.

SPIROCHETES. Spiral-shaped bacteria.

STARI. Southern tick-associated rash illness is a syndrome with unknown causes with symptoms that mimic Lyme disease.

TICK-BORNE RELAPSING FEVER. A tick-borne disease caused by the bacteria *Borrelia miyamotoi, B. hermsii, B. parkeri*, and *B. turicatae*.

TINCTURE. An alcohol extract of dried or fresh plants with medicinal properties.

TULAREMIA. A disease caused by *Francisella tularensis* bacteria. Also known as rabbit fever.

VECTOR. An organism that transmits a disease from one organism to another.

NOTES

1. Tokarz, Rafal, et al., "Microbiome Analysis of Ixodes scapularis Ticks from New York and Connecticut," *Ticks and Tick-Borne Diseases* 10, no. 4 (2019): 894–900, doi:10.1016/j.ttbdis.2019.04.011; *Report of the Other Tick-Borne Diseases and Coinfections Subcommittee to the Tick-Borne Disease Working Group*, Office of the Assistant Secretary for Health, HHS.gov, 2018, www.hhs.gov/ash/advisory-committees/tickbornedisease/reports/other-tbds-2018-5-9/index.html.

2. Edouard Vannier and Peter J. Krause, "Human Babesiosis," *New England Journal of Medicine* 366, no. 25 (June 21, 2012): 2397–2407, doi:10.1056/nejmra1202018.

3. Joy A. Hecht et al., "Multistate Survey of American Dog Ticks (*Dermacentor variabilis*) for *Rickettsia* Species," *Vector-Borne and Zoonotic Diseases* (2019), doi:10.1089/vbz.2018.2415.

4. Melissa Hardstone Yoshimizu and Sarah Billeter, "Suspected and Confirmed Vector-Borne Rickettsioses of North America Associated with Human Diseases," *Tropical Medicine and Infectious Disease* 3, no. 1 (2018): 2, doi:10.3390/tropicalmed3010002.

5. Ellen Y. Stromdahl, Robyn M. Nadolny, Graham J. Hickling, et al., "*Amblyomma americanum* (Acari: Ixodidae) Ticks Are Not Vectors of the Lyme Disease Agent, *Borrelia burgdorferi* (Spirocheatales: Spirochaetaceae): A Review of the Evidence," *Journal of Medical Entomology* 55, no. 3 (May 4, 2018): 501–14, doi:10.1093/jme/tjx250.

6. Stromdahl, "*Amblyomma americanum* (Acari: Ixodidae) Ticks Are Not Vectors."

7. Alejandro Cabezas-Cruz, Pedro J. Espinosa, Pilar Alberdi, et al., "Tick Galactosyltransferases Are Involved in α-Gal Synthesis and Play a Role during *Anaplasma phagocytophilum* Infection and *Ixodes scapularis* Tick Vector Development," *Scientific Reports* 8, no. 1 (September 21, 2018): 14224, doi:10.1038/s41598-018-32664-z.

8. Ben Beard, James Occi, Denise L. Bonilla, et al., "Multistate Infestation with the Exotic Disease–Vector Tick *Haemaphysalis longicornis* — United States, August 2017–September 2018," *Morbidity and Mortality Weekly Report* 67, no. 47 (November 30, 2018): 1310–13, doi:10.15585/mmwr.mm6747a3.

9. Christina A. Nelson, Shubhayu S. Saha, and Paul S. Mead, "Cat-Scratch Disease in the United States, 2005–2013," *Emerging Infectious Diseases* 22. no. 10 (October 2016): 1741–46, doi:10.3201/eid2210.160115.

10. Lucia Pulzova and Mangesh Bhide, "Outer Surface Proteins of *Borrelia*: Peerless Immune Evasion Tools," *Current Protein & Peptide Science* 15, no. 1 (February 2014): 75–88, doi:10.2174/1389203715666140221124213.

11. Kit Tilly, Patricia A. Rosa, and Philip E. Stewart, "Biology of infection with *Borrelia burgdorferi*," *Infectious Disease Clinics of North America* 22, no. 2 (June 2008): 217–34, v, doi:10.1016/j.idc.2007.12.013.

12. Leena Meriläinen, Heini Brander, Anni Herranen, et al., "Pleomorphic Forms of *Borrelia burgdorferi* Induce Distinct Immune Responses," *Microbes and Infection* 18, no. 7–8, (July–August 2016): 484–95, doi:10.1016/j.micinf.2016.04.002.

13. Eva Sapi, "Antimicrobial Resistance of *Borrelia*: Can We Find the Trojan Horse?" Nutramedix 25th Anniversary Meeting, Jupiter, Florida, November 12, 2018.

14. Brian A. Fallon, MD, and Jennifer Sotsky, MD, *Conquering Lyme Disease: Science Bridges the Great Divide* (New York: Columbia University Press, 2018).

15. Holly M. Biggs, Casey Barton Behravesh, Kristy K. Bradley, et al., "Diagnosis and Management of Tickborne Rickettsial Diseases: Rocky Mountain Spotted Fever and Other Spotted Fever Group Rickettsioses, Ehrlichioses, and Anaplasmosis — United States; A Practical Guide for Health Care and Public Health Professionals."

Morbidity and Mortality Weekly Reports: Recommendations and Reports 65, no. 2 (May 2016): 1–44, doi:10.15585/mmwr.rr6502a1.

16. Biggs, "Diagnosis and Management of Tickborne Rickettsial Diseases."

17. Yoshimizu, "Suspected and Confirmed Vector-Borne Rickettsioses of North America."

18. Biggs, "Diagnosis and Management of Tickborne Rickettsial Diseases."

19. Kerry A. Padgett, Denise Bonilla, Marina E. Eremeeva, et al., "The Eco-epidemiology of Pacific Coast Tick Fever in California," *PLoS Neglected Tropical Diseases* 10, no. 10 (October 5, 2016): e0005020, doi:10.1371/journal.pntd.0005020.

20. Meghan E. Hermance and Saravanan Thangamani, "Powassan Virus: An Emerging Arbovirus of Public Health Concern in North America," *Vector Borne and Zoonotic Diseases* 17, no. 7 (July 2017): 453–62, doi:10.1089/vbz.2017.2110.

21. Fallon and Sotsky, *Conquering Lyme Disease*.

22. "Tick-Borne Relapsing Fever," Centers for Disease Control and Prevention, https://www.cdc.gov/relapsing-fever/distribution/index.html. Accessed February 22, 2019.

23. Martin E. Adelson et al., "Prevalence of *Borrelia burgdorferi*, *Bartonella* spp., *Babesia microti*, and *Anaplasma phagocytophila* in *Ixodes scapularis* Ticks Collected in Northern New Jersey," *Journal of Clinical Microbiology* 42, no. 6 (2004): 2799-801, doi:10.1128/JCM.42.6.2799-2801.2004; Kevin Holden et al., "Co-detection of *Bartonella henselae*, *Borrelia burgdorferi*, and *Anaplasma phagocytophilum* in *Ixodes pacificus* Ticks from California, USA," *Vector-Borne and Zoonotic Diseases* 6, no. 1 (2006): 99–102, doi:10.1089/vbz.2006.6.99.

24. Olivier Duron, Karim Sidi-Boumedine, E. Rousset, et al., "The Importance of Ticks in Q Fever Transmission: What Has (and Has Not) Been Demonstrated?," *Trends in Parasitology* 31, no. 11 (November 2015): 536–52, doi:10.1016/j.pt.2015.06.014.

25. Richard S. Ostfeld, *Lyme Disease: The Ecology of a Complex System* (New York: Oxford University Press, 2012).

26. Ostfeld, *Lyme Disease*, 125–26.

27. Scott C. Williams, Megan A. Linske, and Jeffrey S. Ward, "Long-Term Effects of *Berberis thunbergii* (Ranunculales: Berberidaceae) Management on *Ixodes scapularis* (Acari: Ixodidae) Abundance and *Borrelia burgdorferi* (Spirochaetales: Spirochaetaceae) Prevalence in Connecticut, USA," *Environmental Entomology* 46, no. 6 (December 8, 2017): 1329–38, doi:10.1093/ee/nvx146.

28. Megan A. Linske, Scott C. Williams, Jeffrey S. Ward, and Kirby C. Stafford, "Indirect Effects of Japanese Barberry Infestations on White-Footed Mice Exposure to *Borrelia burgdorferi*," *Environmental Entomology* 47, no. 4 (August 11, 2018): 795–802, doi:10.1093/ee/nvy079.

29. Felicia Keesing and Richard S. Ostfeld, "The Tick Project: Testing Environmental Methods of Preventing Tick-Borne Diseases," *Trends in Parasitology* 34, no. 6 (June 2018): 447–50, doi:10.1016/j.pt.2018.03.005.

30. Kirby C. Stafford and Sandra A. Allan, "Field Applications of Entomopathogenic Fungi *Beauveria bassiana* and *Metarhizium anisopliae* F52 (Hypocreales: Clavicipitaceae) for the Control of *Ixodes scapularis* (Acari: Ixodidae)," *Journal of Medical Entomology* 47, no. 6 (November 2010): 1107–15, doi:10.1603/me10019.

31. Catherine Regnault-Roger, "The Potential of Botanical Essential Oils for Insect Pest Control," *Integrated Pest Management Reviews* 2, no. 1 (February 1997): 25–34, doi:10.1016/j.jep.2016.11.002.

32. Ostfeld, *Lyme Disease*.

33. "Damminix Tick Tubes Test Results on Fire Island, N.Y.," Ecohealth Inc., www.ticktubes.com/downloads/ticktubes_fire_island_study.pdf. Accessed March 11, 2018.

34. Erin C. Jones, Alison F. Hinckley, Sarah A. Hook, et al., "Pet Ownership Increases Human Risk of Encountering Ticks," *Zoonoses and Public Health* 65, no. 1 (February 2018): 74–79, doi:10.1111/zph.12369.

35. "Protect Your Pets — Tick Control on Pets," TickEncounter Resource Center, www .tickencounter.org/prevention/tick_control#top. Accessed February 10, 2019.

36. Christina A. Nelson et al., "The Heat Is On: Killing Blacklegged Ticks in Residential Washers and Dryers to Prevent Tickborne Diseases," *Ticks and Tick-Borne Diseases* 7, no. 5 (2016): 958–63, doi:10.1016/j.ttbdis.2016.04.016.

37. Jennifer Hostetler, *Laboratory Bioassay to Assess the Repellency and Efficacy of One Direct Spray Product against Multiple Species, in Terms of Knockdown and Mortality*, i2LResearch USA, Inc., July 2018.

38. Gabrielle Dietrich, Marc C. Dolan, Javier Peralta-Cruz, et al., "Repellent Activity of Fractioned Compounds from *Chamaecyparis nootkatensis* Essential Oil against Nymphal *Ixodes scapularis* (Acari: Ixodidae)," *Journal of Medical Entomology* 43, no. 5 (January 2006): 957–61, doi:10.1603/0022-2585(2006)43[957: raofcf]2.0.co;2.

39. Robert A. Jordan, Terry L. Schulze, and Marc C. Dolan, "Efficacy of Plant-Derived and Synthetic Compounds on Clothing as Repellents against *Ixodes scapularis* and *Amblyomma americanum* (Acari: Ixodidae)," *Journal of Medical Entomology* 49, no. 1 (January 2012): 101–6, https://doi.org/10.1603/ME10241.

40. Nathan J. Miller, Erin E. Rainone, Megan C. Dyer, and Liliana Gonzalez, "Tick Bite Protection with Permethrin-Treated Summer-Weight Clothing," *Journal of Medical Entomology* 48, no. 2 (January 2011): 327–33, doi:10.1603/me10158.

41. "Permethrin Insect Repellent Treatment for Clothing Gear and Tents," Sawyer Products, sawyer.com/products/ permethrin-insect-repellent-treatment/.

42. "Knockdown Testing," Insect Shield, www.insectshield.com/Knockdown-Testing.aspx. Accessed March 11, 2018.

43. Meagan F. Vaughn and Steven R. Meshnick, "Pilot Study Assessing the Effectiveness of Long-Lasting Permethrin-Impregnated Clothing for the Prevention of Tick Bites," *Vector-Borne and Zoonotic Diseases* 11, no. 7 (July 2011): 869–75, doi:10.1089/vbz.2010.0158.

44. "Scent Recognition," Insect Shield, www.insectshield.com/Scent-Recognition.aspx. Accessed March 11, 2018.

45. Robert B. Nadelman et al., "Prophylaxis with Single-Dose Doxycycline for the Prevention of Lyme Disease after *Anixodes scapularis* Tick Bite," *New England Journal of Medicine* 345, no. 2 (2001): 79–84, doi:10.1056/ nejm200107123450201.

46. Stephen Y. Gbedema et al., "Antimalarial Activity of *Cryptolepis sanguinolenta* Based Herbal Capsules in *Plasmodium berghei* Infected Mice," *International Research Journal in Phamacy* 2, no. 5 (2011): 127–31.

47. Stephen Harrod Buhner, *Herbal Antivirals: Natural Remedies for Emerging Resistant and Epidemic Viral Infections* (North Adams, MA: Storey Publishing, 2013).

48. Stephanie Richards, Ricky Langley, Charles Apperson, and Elizabeth Watson, "Do Tick Attachment Times Vary between Different Tick-Pathogen Systems?," *Environments* no. 2 (September 2017): 37, doi:10.3390/ environments4020037.

49. Chien-Ming Shih and Andrew Spielman. "Accelerated Transmission of Lyme Disease Spirochetes by Partially Fed Vector Ticks," *Journal of Clinical Microbiology* 31, no. 11 (November 1993): 2878–81.

50. Shih, "Accelerated Transmission of Lyme Disease."

51. Lars Eisen, "Pathogen Transmission in Relation to Duration of Attachment by *Ixodes* *scapularis* Ticks," *Ticks and Tick-Borne Diseases* 9, no. 3 (March 2018): 535–42, doi:10.1016/j.ttbdis.2018.01.002.

52. Daniel J. Cameron, Lorraine B. Johnson, and Elizabeth L. Maloney, "Evidence Assessments and Guideline Recommendations in Lyme Disease: The Clinical Management of Known Tick Bites, Erythema Migrans Rashes and Persistent Disease," *Expert Review of Anti-infective Therapy* 12, no. 9 (September 2014): 1103–35, doi:10.1586/14787210.2014.940900.

53. Fallon and Sotsky, *Conquering Lyme Disease*, p. 83.

54. F. Breier et al., "Isolation and Polymerase Chain Reaction Typing of *Borrelia afzelii* from a Skin Lesion in a Seronegative Patient with Generalized Ulcerating Bullous Lichen Sclerosus et Atrophicus," *British Journal of Dermatology* 144, no. 2 (2001): 387–92, doi:10.1046/j.1365-2133.2001.04034.x. Michael Brunner, "New Method for Detection of *Borrelia burgdorferi* Antigen Complexed to Antibody in Seronegative Lyme Disease," *Journal of Immunological Methods* 249, no. 1–2 (2001): 185–90, doi:10.1016/s0022-1759(00)00356-2. P. Coulter et al., "Two-Year Evaluation of *Borrelia burgdorferi* Culture and Supplemental Tests for Definitive Diagnosis of Lyme Disease," *Journal of Clinical Microbiology* 43, no. 10 (January 2005): 5080–84, doi:10.1128/jcm.43.10.5080-5084.2005. H. Dejmková et al., "Seronegative Lyme Arthritis Caused by *Borrelia garinii*," *Clinical Rheumatology* 21, no. 4, (2002): 330–34, doi:10.1007/s100670200087. Reinhard Kaiser, "False-Negative Serology in Patients with Neuroborreliosis and the Value of Employing of Different Borrelial Strains in Serological Assays," *Journal of Medical Microbiology* 49, no. 10 (January 2000): 911–15, doi:10.1099/0022-1317-49-10-911. A. Marangoni, "Comparative Evaluation of Three Different ELISA Methods for the Diagnosis of Early Culture-Confirmed Lyme Disease in Italy," *Journal of Medical Microbiology* 54, no. 4 (January 2005): 361–67, doi:10.1099/

jmm.0.45853-0. Franjo Pikelji, "Seronegative Lyme Disease and Transitory Atrioventricular Block," *Annals of Internal Medicine* 111, no. 1 (January 1989): 90, doi:10.7326/0003-4819-111-1-90_1. S. E. Schutzer et al., "Sequestration of Antibody to *Borrelia burgdorferi* in Immune Complexes in Seronegative Lyme Disease," *Lancet* 335, no. 8685 (1990): 312–15. Allen Steere, "Seronegative Lyme Disease," *JAMA: The Journal of the American Medical Association* 270, no. 11 (October 1993): 1369, doi:10.1001/jama.1993.03510110111042. Iwona Wojciechowska-Koszko et al., "Serodiagnosis of Borreliosis: Indirect Immunofluorescence Assay, Enzyme-Linked Immunosorbent Assay and Immunoblotting," *Archivum Immunologiae et Therapiae Experimentalis* 59, no. 1 (February 2011): 69–77, doi:10.1007/s00005-010-0111-0.

55. "Lyme ImmunoBlot IgM and IgG," IGeneX Inc., https://igenex.com/wp-content/uploads/LymeImmunoBlot-DataSheet.pdf. Accessed January 9, 2018.

56. US Centers for Disease Control and Prevention, "Rocky Mountain Spotted Fever: Treatment," https://www.cdc.gov/rmsf/healthcare-providers/treatment.html. Accessed June 10, 2019.

57. M. Dinleyici and Y. Vandenplas, "*Clostridium difficile* Colitis Prevention and Treatment," *Advances in Experimental Medicine and Biology*. New York: Springer, 2019.

58. For more information on the two sets of guidelines, see Lorraine Johnson, "Two Standards of Care in Lyme Disease," on the LymeDisease.org website, https://www.lymedisease.org/wp-content/uploads/2015/01/2014-Two-Standards-of-Care-Revisited-1.7.15-FINAL.pdf. Accessed May 7, 2019.

RESOURCES

LYME-LITERATE PRACTITIONERS

To find a Lyme-literate practitioner, consult any of the following organizations, which are dedicated to Lyme and tick-borne disease education, advocacy, and research.

Global Lyme Alliance
https://globallymealliance.org/

International Lyme and Associated Diseases Society (ILADS)
https://www.ilads.org/

LymeDisease.org
https://www.lymedisease.org/

TESTING FOR TICKS AND TICK-BORNE DISEASES

IGeneX Inc.
www.igenex.com
IGeneX is one of the leaders in developing ever more sensitive tests for Lyme and other tick-borne diseases. This lab allows you to work with your medical practitioner to order appropriate diagnostic blood tests.

Medical Diagnostic Laboratories
www.mdlab.com
Medical Diagnostic Laboratories is a specialty laboratory that offers tests for tick-borne diseases. This lab allows you to work with your medical practitioner to order appropriate diagnostic blood tests.

TickReport
www.tickreport.com
TickReport uses highly specific, highly sensitive qPCR testing that detects the DNA or RNA of pathogens in a tick. It can test for a wide range of tick pathogens and sends out results within 3 business days. The lab keeps ticks indefinitely so a customer may request testing for other pathogens at a later date.

TICK-RELATED GEAR AND SUPPLIES

Cedarcide
www.cedarcide.com
Cedarcide makes a variety of natural insect repellents, including Tickshield, based on cedar oil, which has been proven to repel ticks.

Ecohealth, Inc.
www.ticktubes.com
Supplier of Damminix Tick Tubes; order online or find out where you can purchase them locally.

Insect Shield
www.insectshield.com
Send your clothing to Insect Shield for a long-lasting tick-repellent permethrin treatment.

NootkaShield
www.evolva.com/nootkashield
This nootkatone-based "biopesticide" has been shown to be highly effective against ticks. Check this website for its release date; the product is currently under government review.

O'Tom
www.otom.com
Supplier of Tick Twister by O'Tom, a tick removal tool.

Thermacell
www.thermacell.com
Supplier of Thermacell Tick Control Tubes, which you can order online.

Tick Box Technology Corporation
www.tickboxtcs.com
Supplier of Tick Box Tick Control Systems; the website can direct you to a certified local installer.

HERBS, HOMEOPATHIC REMEDIES, AND SUPPLEMENTS

Blue Crow Botanicals
www.bluecrowbotanicals.com
Offers a wide range of single-herb tinctures and multi-herb formulas, including the very same deer tick bite formula I use with my patients and describe in this book. Also offers fresh *Houttuynia cordata* plants, if you're in the area of western Massachusetts.

Boiron
www.boironusa.com
Offers homeopathic remedies like *Ledum* and *Apis*, which are recommended as part of the first-aid response to a tick bite.

Healing Spirits Herb Farm and Education Center
www.healingspiritsherbfarm.com
Offers a wide range of herbs and tinctures, including the highest-quality Japanese knotweed root currently available in North America. Contact them via the website's contact form or by calling 607-566-2701.

Herbie's Herbs

www.herbies-herbs.com

Offers all of the herbs called for in the formulas in this book, as dried herbs or tinctures. At the time of writing this book, it is the only trusted source for dried cryptolepis in North America.

Mountain Rose Herbs

www.mountainroseherbs.com

Offers many of the herbs called for in the formulas in this book, as dried herbs or tinctures, including dried *Uncaria tomentosa* (cat's claw) bark. Mountain Rose Herbs uses sustainable, fair-trade practices.

Nutramedix

www.nutramedix.com

Offers high-quality, physician-grade, third party–tested herbal medicines and supplements used to treat Lyme and tick-borne disease. It carries all of the products used in the prophylactic deer tick bite protocol designed for children (page 98): houttuynia, Mora, Samento, and serrapeptase.

Sojourns Community Health Clinic

www.sojourns.org

Sojourns Community Health Clinic is a nonprofit integrative health clinic in southern Vermont. Sojourns has a client-centered approach and is committed to education, community outreach, and economic accessibility. Sojourns' innovative health-care model offers over a dozen practitioners in a variety of disciplines who work together.

The Apothecary at Sojourns Community Health Clinic offers a wide variety of high-quality products, including vitamins, supplements, homeopathic remedies, dried herbs, tinctures, essential oils, flower essences, and natural living products. All of the single-herb tinctures, multi-herb formulas, and supplements (including serrapeptase) mentioned in this book are available. Anyone may visit the Apothecary in person or call to place an order for shipment.

Strictly Medicinal Seeds

www.strictlymedicinalseeds.com

Can ship fresh houttuynia plants directly to your doorstep. Note that houttuynia can be found via the website under the name "chameleon plant."

Woodland Essence

www.woodlandessence.com

Offers all of the single-herb tinctures called for in the formulas in this book, as organic or wild-crafted. They also carry many glycerites, which serve as an alternative to tinctures for those who are sensitive to alcohol.

INFORMATION

For more information on ticks, Lyme, and other tick-borne diseases, and for current treatment options, consult any of the following organizations.

Bay Area Lyme Foundation
www.bayarealyme.org

Canadian Lyme Disease Foundation
https://canlyme.com

Caring for & Healing
www.caringforandhealing.com
This site, the creation of the parent of a child with Lyme, offers an eight-step framework of care for parents and caretakers of children with Lyme and other tick-borne disease, disability, or chronic illness, some of which may be applied to adults.

Children's Lyme Disease Network
www.childrenslymenetwork.org

Columbia University Irving Lyme and Tick-Borne Diseases Research Center
www.columbia-lyme.org

Global Lyme Alliance
www.gla.org

International Lyme and Associated Diseases Society (ILADS)
www.ilads.org

Lyme Disease Association, Inc.
https://lymediseaseassociation.org

LymeDisease.org
www.lymedisease.org

The National Capital Lyme Disease Association
www.natcaplyme.org

PA (Pennsylvania) Lyme Resource Network
https://palyme.org

Tick-Borne Disease Working Group
The Tick-Borne Disease Working Group was established by the 2016 21st Century Cures Act to improve federal coordination of efforts related to tick-borne diseases. Members will review all U.S. Department of Health and Human Services efforts related to tick-borne diseases to provide expertise and "help ensure interagency coordination and minimize overlap, examine research priorities," and identify unmet needs.
To read the *Tick-Borne Disease Working Group 2018 Report to Congress:* **https://www.hhs.gov/sites/default/files/tbdwg-report-to-congress-2018.pdf**

To participate in meetings and public comment periods and read future reports: **https://www.hhs.gov/ash/advisory-committees/tickbornedisease/index.html**

TickEncounter Resource Center
www.tickencounter.org
The TickEncounter Resource Center at
the University of Rhode Island offers
excellent information on tick bite and
tick-borne disease prevention. This
highly interactive website offers endless resources in the form of photos
and videos as well as TickSmart learning kits available for purchase.

VTLyme.org (in Vermont)
www.VTLyme.org

SUPPORT GROUPS

LymeDisease.org
www.lymedisease.org
Offers an online listing of state-based
Lyme support groups; click on the "Get
Involved" tab on the group's main page.

RawlsMD Lyme Support Directory
https://rawlsmd.com/lyme-support
Offers a database of Lyme support
groups.

FINANCIAL AID

Lyme Light Foundation
www.lymelightfoundation.org
Financial assistance for the treatment of
Lyme and TBD patients through age 25.

Lyme Test Access Program
www.lymetap.com
Financial assistance for Lyme-related
laboratory testing for patients.

Ticked Off Foundation
www.tickedofffoundation.org
Maintains a financial assistance fund
for Lyme and TBD patients 26 years
and older.

FOR FURTHER READING

The Beginner's Guide to Lyme Disease: Diagnosis and Treatment Made Simple, by Nicola McFadzean, ND

Conquering Lyme Disease: Science Bridges the Great Divide, by Brian A. Fallon, MD, and Jennifer Sotsky, MD

Cure Unknown: Inside the Lyme Epidemic, by Pamela Weintraub

Healing Lyme Disease Coinfections: Complementary and Holistic Treatments for Bartonella and Mycoplasma, by Stephen Harrod Buhner

Healing Lyme: Natural Healing of Lyme Borreliosis and the Coinfections Chlamydia and Spotted Fever Rickettsiosis, 2nd edition, by Stephen Harrod Buhner

Herbal Antivirals: Natural Remedies for Emerging & Resistant Viral Infections, by Stephen Harrod Buhner

How Can I Get Better? An Action Plan for Treating Resistant Lyme and Chronic Disease, by Richard I. Horowitz, MD

Living beyond Lyme: Reclaim Your Life from Lyme Disease and Chronic Illness, by Joseph J. Trunzo, PhD

The Lyme Diet: Nutritional Strategies for Healing from Lyme Disease, by Nicola McFadzean, ND

The Lyme Disease Solution, by Kenneth Singleton, MD, MPH

The Lyme Solution: A 5-Point Plan to Fight the Inflammatory Auto-immune Response and Beat Lyme Disease, by Darin Ingels, ND, FAAEM

Natural Treatments for Lyme Coinfections: Anaplasma, Babesia, and Ehrlichia, by Stephen Harrod Buhner

New Paradigms in Lyme Disease Treatment: 10 Top Doctors Reveal Healing Strategies That Work, by Connie Strasheim

Recipes for Repair: A Lyme Disease Cookbook, by Gail Piazza and Laura Piazza

Rising Above Lyme Disease: A Revolutionary, Holistic Approach to Managing and Reversing the Symptoms of Lyme Disease — And Reclaiming Your Life, by Julia Greenspan, ND

Toxic: Heal Your Body from Mold Toxicity, Lyme Disease, Multiple Chemical Sensitivities, and Chronic Environmental Illness, by Neil Nathan, MD

When Your Child Has Lyme Disease: A Parent's Survival Guide, by Sandra K. Berenbaum and Dorothy Kupcha Leland

Why Can't I Get Better? Solving the Mystery of Lyme and Chronic Disease, by Richard I. Horowitz, MD

INDEX

Page numbers in *italic* indicate illustrations; numbers in **bold** indicate charts.

immune system and, 43

mammal host and, 38–39

proteins and, 37–38

round body forms, 39–40, *39*

spirochete classification, 37

treatment protocol for, 149–150

Borrelia hermsii, 6

Borrelia species, as atypical bacterium, 37–39

borreliosis, 40. *See also* Lyme disease

brown dog tick, 24, 25

tick-borne pathogens and, 141

Brown Dog Tick Bite Formula, 94

Buhner, Stephen, 158

bull's eye rash. *See* erythema migrans

Burgdorfer, Willy, 36

C

candidiasis (yeast overgrowth), 163

case study, testing after deer tick bite, 141–43

cat's claw. *See Uncaria rhynchophylla, U. tomentosa*

C. diff (Clostridioides difficile), 163

cefuroxime, 161

children

adjusting dosages for, 99

prophylactic protocols for, 98–99

ciprofloxacin, 162

clothing. *See* tick-repellent clothing

coinfections, 6, 10

Colorado tick fever, *57*

acute, treatment for, 158

signs and symptoms, 57

Cordyceps militaris, C. sinensis (cordyceps), 110, *110*

Coxiella burnetii, 61

Cryptolepis sanguinolenta (cryptolepsis), 111, *111*

cytokines, 39

D

dan shen. *See Salvia miltiorrhiza*

deer-resistant plants, 74–75

deer tick. *See* blacklegged tick

deer tick bite, testing case study, 141–43

Deer Tick Bite Formula, 91

for children, 98–99

Deer Tick Bite Prophylactic Formula, 102

combining tinctures, 106

tincturing dried herbs, 103–4

tincturing fresh herbs, 105–6

deer tick-borne disease, 45

direct agglutination (DA) technique, 136

direct testing, tick bites and, 137

disease(s). *See* tick-borne diseases; *specific disease*

disease treatment, acute tick-borne, 144–159

beginning treatment, 147–48

Lyme disease, 148–150

protocol, nonpregnant adult, 149–150

dorsal shield (scutum), 28, *28*

doxycycline, 85, 148, 149, 161

E

educational resource, 31

ehrlichiosis, *47*

acute, treatment for, 152

rash resulting from, 133–34

signs and symptoms, 47–48

ELISA (enzyme-linked immunosorbent assay) technique, 136, 142

enzyme, prophylaxis and, 119

erythema migrans (rash), 133

bull's eye, 9–10, 43

characteristics, 42, 146

disseminated, 42

doxycycline and, 85

patterns, 43

essential oils, 69–70

Take Good Care, Naturally, with More Books from Storey

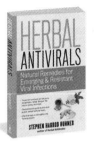

Herbal Antivirals
BY STEPHEN HARROD BUHNER
Boost your immune system with this complete guide to the most potent natural antiviral herbs. Prepare and use herbal formulas to fight against viral infections from the flu to encephalitis, Ebola, and much more.

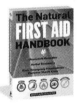

The Natural First Aid Handbook, 2nd Edition BY BRIGITTE MARS
Be prepared to handle those critical first moments after an injury or the onset of illness. Effective herbal and homeopathic remedies, along with basic first aid techniques and survival skills, arm you with the know-how you need when you're far from immediate help.

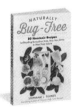

Naturally Bug-Free BY STEPHANIE L. TOURLES
Protect yourself from mosquitoes, ticks, and other biting insects without relying on chemicals. These 75 all-natural recipes for sprays, balms, body oils, and tinctures — plus herbal pet shampoos, flea collars, and powders — are safe for your body, pets, and home.

Join the conversation. Share your experience with this book, learn more about Storey Publishing's authors, and read original essays and book excerpts at storey.com. Look for our books wherever quality books are sold or call 800-441-5700.

◎ TICK ID

Use the guide below to help identify your tick. Pay special attention to the scutum.

BLACKLEGGED TICK

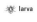 larva
 nymph

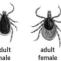
adult male   adult female

partially fed

scutum

engorged

WESTERN BLACKLEGGED TICK

 larva
 nymph

adult male   adult female

scutum

partially fed

engorged

AMERICAN DOG TICK

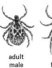 larva
 nymph

adult male   adult female

scutum

partially fed

engorged

LONE STAR TICK

 larva
 nymph

adult male   adult female

scutum

partially fed

engorged

◎ TICK ID

Here we have ticks at their actual (average) size. Keep this card with you to help you make a positive identification of any ticks you find.

5 mm   10 mm   15 mm   20 mm

	BLACKLEGGED TICK (deer tick)	WESTERN BLACKLEGGED TICK (deer tick)	AMERICAN DOG TICK
larva (left) nymph (right)			
adult male (left) adult female (right)	2.5 mm	2.5 mm	5.0 mm
scutum			
partially fed (left) engorged (right)	10 mm (max)	10 mm (max)	15 mm (max)

◎ TICK ID

Here we have ticks at their actual (average) size. Keep this card with you to help you make a positive identification of any ticks you find.

5 mm   10 mm   15 mm   20 mm

	BLACKLEGGED TICK (deer tick)	WESTERN BLACKLEGGED TICK (deer tick)	AMERICAN DOG TICK
larva (left) nymph (right)			
adult male (left) adult female (right)	2.5 mm	2.5 mm	5.0 mm
scutum			
partially fed (left) engorged (right)	10 mm (max)	10 mm (max)	15 mm (max)

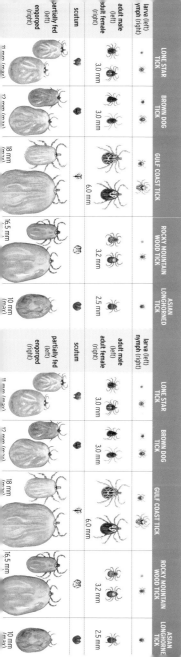

	LONE STAR TICK	BROWN DOG TICK	GULF COAST TICK	ROCKY MOUNTAIN WOOD TICK	ASIAN LONGHORNED TICK
larva (left) nymph (right)	*	*	*	*	*
adult male (left) adult female (right)	3.0 mm	3.0 mm	6.0 mm	3.2 mm	2.5 mm
scutum					
partially fed (left) engorged (right)	11 mm (max)	12 mm (max)	18 mm (max)	16.5 mm	10 mm (max)

	LONE STAR TICK	BROWN DOG TICK	GULF COAST TICK	ROCKY MOUNTAIN WOOD TICK	ASIAN LONGHORNE TICK
larva (left) nymph (right)	*	*	*	*	*
adult male (left) adult female (right)	3.0 mm	3.0 mm	6.0 mm	3.2 mm	2.5 mm
scutum					
partially fed (left) engorged (right)	11 mm (max)	12 mm (max)	18 mm (max)	16.5 mm	10 mm (max)

BROWN DOG TICK

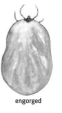

larva

nymph

adult male

adult female

partially fed

scutum

engorged

GULF COAST TICK

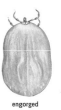

larva

nymph

adult male

adult female

partially fed

scutum

engorged

ROCKY MOUNTAIN WOOD TICK

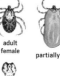

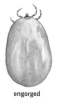

larva

nymph

adult male

adult female

partially fed

scutum

engorged

ASIAN LONGHORNED TICK

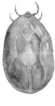

nymph

adult

scutum

engorged

ORNITHODOROS TICK (5 to 7 mm long)

O. hermsi

O. turicata

O. parkeri

THE LYME RASH

Erythema migrans, the rash caused by Lyme disease, can manifest in many ways. Most familiar is the classic bull's-eye lesion, with the tick bite in the center. However, the color, shape, and borders vary, as you can see by the examples shown here.

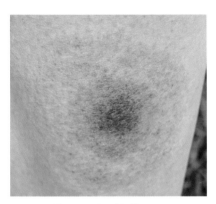

Classic bull's-eye rash, with discrete outer border and partial central clearing

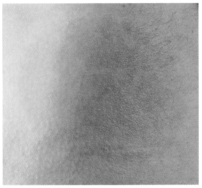

Circular, uniformly red-pink rash

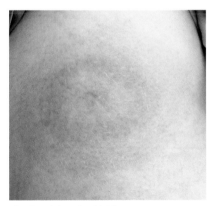

Circular pink rash with blue center.

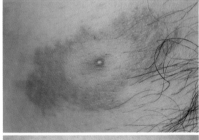

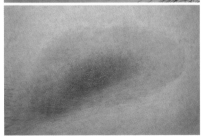

Oval or elliptical rash with irregular borders

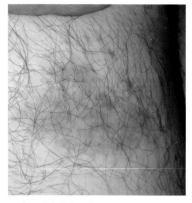

Lesion with diffuse borders

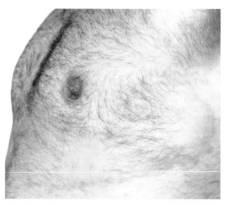

Larger lesion with discrete yet hard-to-see borders

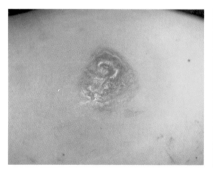

Bullous rash, with a large blister

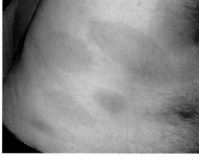

Disseminated rash, with lesions in multiple locations